THE TV VET BOOK
FOR STOCK FARMERS NO. 2

THE TV VET BOOK
FOR STOCK FARMERS NO. 2

Calving the Cow
and Care of the Calf

By
THE TV VET

FARMING PRESS LTD
FENTON HOUSE WHARFEDALE ROAD IPSWICH SUFFOLK

TV Vet Book for Stock Farmers

FIRST PUBLISHED 1965
SECOND EDITION 1972
SECOND IMPRESSION 1973
THIRD IMPRESSION 1974
FOURTH IMPRESSION 1976
FIFTH IMPRESSION 1977

ISBN 0 85236 011 8

This book is set in 'Monophoto' Times 10pt on 11pt and is printed in Great Britain by
Cox & Wyman Ltd, London, Fakenham and Reading

Contents

CARE OF THE CALF

Foreword

By JOHN CHERRINGTON

MANY years ago I was working on a farm in New Zealand. One of our house cows developed what I now know to be milk fever, but to us the illness was a mystery. Being fresh from England, I said to the boss: "Shall I get the vet?" To which he replied: "Don't talk nonsense boy, a vet costs money, cut its ruddy throat, we'll feed it to the dogs."

Times have changed now and a vet's bill is usually a better investment than the knackerman's cheque. But like many farmers I like to know what is going on, even if I prefer to let the vet do the dirty work for me.

In this book the TV Vet shows in clear photograph and simple text all the problems, and their solutions, to be found when calving cows and rearing calves.

I learned my animal midwifery the hard way by practical experience, and it was particularly hard on the animals, I fear. There is no substitute for practical experience, but with this book to help him, any young farmer and—dare I say it—veterinary surgeon, too, will be greatly helped in understanding symptoms and effecting cures. I wish it well.

Tangley,   JOHN CHERRINGTON
Near Andover,
Hampshire

To the memory of the late Hilary Phillips,
Producer of B.B.C. TV 'Farming',
whose brilliant mind inspired all who had the
privilege of knowing him.

Author's Preface

THIS is 'it'—a concise catalogue of all the invaluable commonsense practical facts concerning calving and calves which I have learned the hard way throughout my career in veterinary practice. Nothing is written from theory—only from personal observation and practical experience, and I'm sure everyone will agree that there is no substitute for experience.

I have made full use of the visual aids but this time, because of the more specific text, the illustrations are vitally important.

The intelligent stockman and farmer should find many useful hints but the student, by taking full note of everything portrayed, will save himself many hours of heartache and frustration. When I was a student, I would have given anything for even a photograph of a prolapsed uterus. To be provided with a comprehensive galaxy of vital practical illustrations would have been little short of miraculous.

I am certain that all farmers, stockmen, students and younger veterinary surgeons will find this volume of inestimable value.

Two other important points—nearly one third of all losses in cattle are associated with calving and calf conditions, and practically all the material contained in this volume is applicable to the cattle and calves in every part of the world.

Again I would like to pay tribute to my photographer, Mr George Pringle, who is responsible for all the pictures—many of them taken at queer times and in the most awkward situations.

I should like also to thank my colleaques in the features department of the *Farmer & Stockbreeder*, who impressed upon me the value of the 'photo-feature'. And all the farmers who have co-operated in the taking of the pictures, especially Mr Thacker, the owner and manufacturer of the ideal calf pens and hospital boxes, who built his hospital box exactly to my specification.

CALVING THE COW

1
Natural Birth

FOR some time now I have been campaigning in both the veterinary and farming worlds for a more rational approach to the calving of heifers and cows.

Frankly, I am astonished that the strong-arm tactics of pulling the calf like a cork from a bottle ever came into being in an enlightened country. Reflect for a moment on the breeding conditions of animals in the wild state and you will realize just how stupid such methods are.

Of course nature is not completely infallible, and there are times when assistance with calving is necessary, but such occasions are few. I would say without doubt that, provided the foetus is straight—and I repeat this, only when the foetus is straight—the vast majority of animals will give birth naturally if they are given a reasonable chance to do so.

It is vitally important, therefore, before ever attempting to assist at calving time, to have a thorough knowledge of the simple natural birth or, in other words, to really understand the job. *(Below.)*

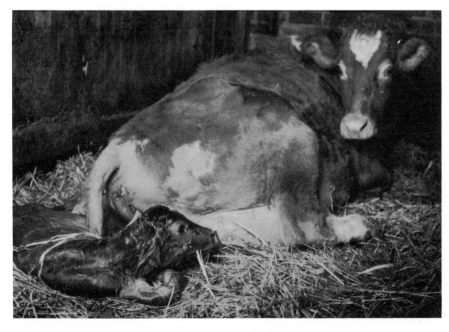

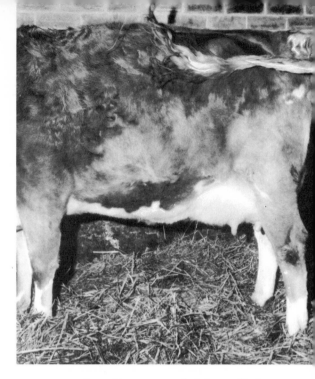

There are three stages in the natural birth *the first or preliminary stage, the second stage,* and *the third or final stage.*

When the heifer first starts 'fairing' for calving, and throughout the whole of the preliminary stage, she shows signs of intermittent uneasiness and slight pain. This despite the fact that she may eat, drink and behave perfectly normally in every way. In fact, throughout the whole of this preliminary phase the animal is bright and cheerful and fully aware of everything going on around her.

The same, of course, holds good in humans—all through the first stage in human labour the patient will eat, drink and chat normally to her friends. Just one difference—where a woman may want to sit or lie back, the heifer or cow stays on her feet all through the first stage.

The first sign is usually an angry swish of the tail and a restless forward movement. *(Top, right.)* She will move forward in a clockwise or anticlockwise semi-circle, very often alternating the one direction with the other. If she is tied up, she will keep moving sharply over in her stall or turning her head to look towards her hind end. Occasionally she may kick at her belly.

These initial spasms of uneasiness occur every 4 or 5 minutes and last only for about 3 to 5 seconds.

What exactly is happening inside at this stage? Each time the muscular wall of the uterus (womb) contracts in labour *(below, left)*, the animal feels a slight, sharp pain —this produces her uneasiness.

At the same time the wave of contraction, which extends throughout the entire womb muscle, causes the so-called water-bladder, which surrounds the foetus, to press against and open up the cervix or entrance to the uterus. *(Below.)* The precise mechanism of this 'opening up' or 'dilation' is not fully understood, but it appears to be due to reflex stimulation, triggered

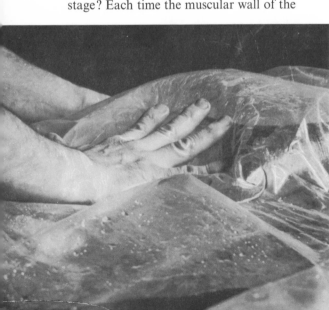

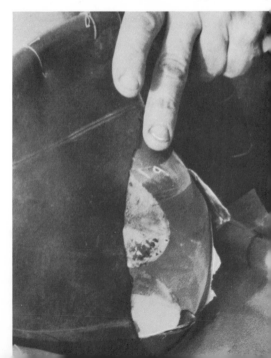

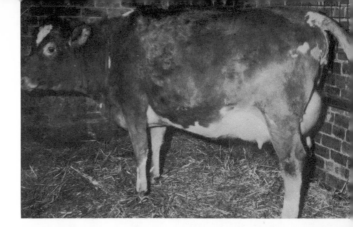

off by the intermittent pressure and relaxation of the water-bladder caused by the uterine contractions.

As the first stage progresses, the uterine contractions become marked enough to cause the animal to arch her back and strain slightly. *(Top, right.)* The first strains usually occur at intervals of three to four minutes and the actual strain lasts only for one second, though the back may remain arched and the tail cocked for between 5 and 10 seconds.

Inside the patient, the uterine contractions are now distinctly stronger and more frequent. The cervix is dilating progressively. *(Below.)*

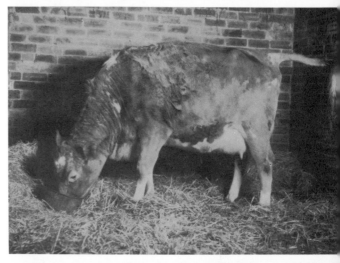

Despite this increased straining, the patient will continue to behave normally, eating and drinking and being fully aware of everything around her. *(Centre, right.)*

However, there are two marked changes, both indicative of the pain of her labour. First of all, her breathing becomes much more rapid—about twice the normal rate—and, secondly, during the uterine contraction, the muscles of the brisket, neck and head region shiver and twitch markedly.

Towards the end of the preliminary labour, the straining bouts become more frequent and each bout comprises several

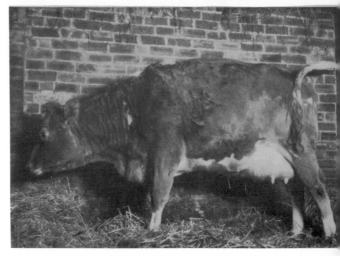

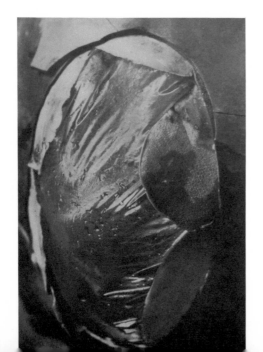

perceptible but mild strains. *(Above.)*

All this while, of course, the patient is standing up and/or walking round in alternate clockwise and anti-clockwise

15

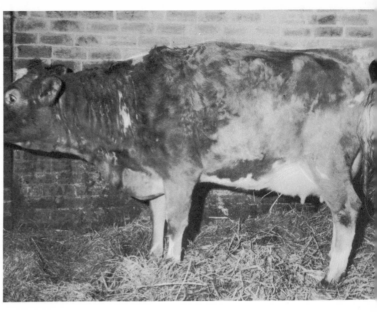

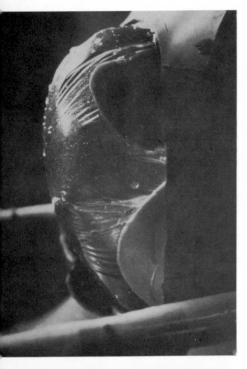

semi-circles. During the last hour of this first-stage labour, the bouts of straining occur approximately every 1½ to 3 minutes and the number of perceptible strains in each varies from one to a dozen or more.

Inside the mother, the cervix is now almost three-quarters dilated and the water-bladder is starting to balloon through the opening. (Top, left.) Up to this stage, the dilation of the cervix is entirely dependent on the water-bladder pressure.

The strains will be seen to get stronger and stronger, and during the last few efforts before the end of the preliminary stage copious urine and dung are passed. (Top, right.) This is nature's way of making certain that as much room as possible will be available for the passage of the calf down the vagina.

Finally, at the end of the first stage in labour, the pains of the uterine contractions make the cow lie down. (Left.)

This preliminary stage lasts for an average of 2 to 3 hours in a cow and 4 to 6 hours in a heifer, though I have seen it continue quite normally for very much longer than that. This is not altogether surprising when one realises that the preliminary stage in women can last quite normally for up to 20 hours. In the heifer

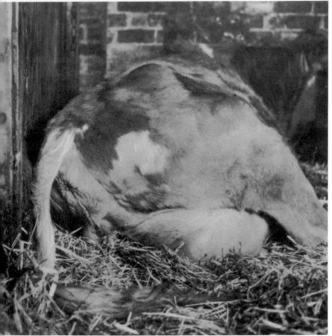

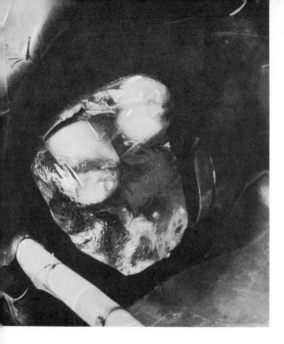

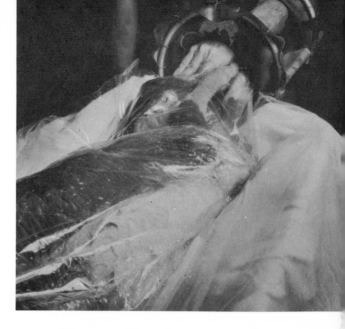

photographed, preliminary labour lasted for exactly 5 hours.

Inside the heifer, the cervix is now three-quarters dilated. A portion of the water-bladder is through into the anterior vagina and the feet of the calf are also poking through the cervix. (Above, left.)

Another interesting and important feature here—the feet are presented sideways. Further careful exploration will show that the calf is actually lying on its left side, with the left cheek of the head resting on the floor of the uterine body. (Above, right.)

The potential mother now goes into second-stage labour which, as in humans, is a very much more serious and intense affair.

The character of the patient changes markedly. Instead of being bright, lively and taking full notice, she appears to become oblivious of her surroundings and concentrates on her intense 'bearing down'. (Below.) This again has an analogy in women, where the character changes markedly—the women behave abnormally and take no heed whatsoever if someone speaks to them.

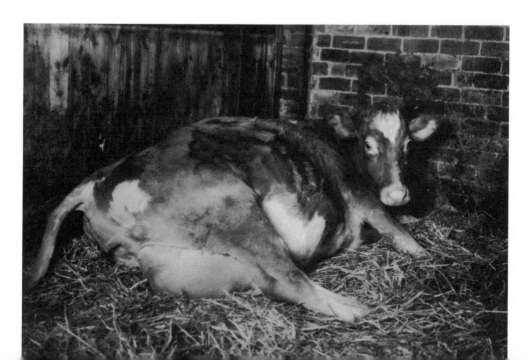

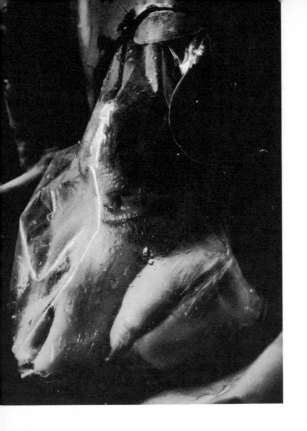

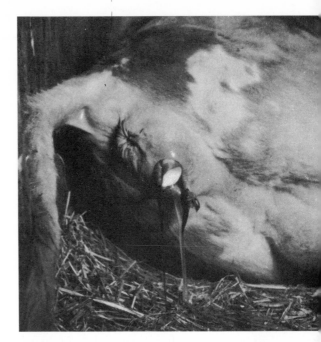

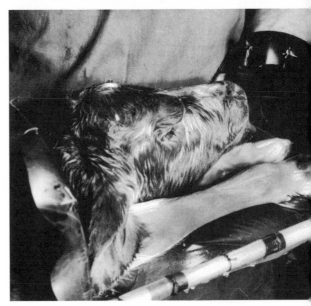

In the heifer, the intervals between the bouts of labour still vary from $1\frac{1}{2}$ to $2\frac{1}{2}$ to even $3\frac{1}{2}$ minutes, but the bouts now comprise really vigorous strains each of which last from $\frac{1}{2}$ to $1\frac{1}{2}$ seconds.

After about a dozen of these severe strains of second-stage labour, and during this time, the calf rotates to its normal correct horizontal position—i.e., it rotates through $\frac{1}{4}$ circle in an anti-clockwise direction. From now on, each strain causes the top of the calf's head to bear on the top inside of the cervix, and this renewed intermittent pressure causes the cervix to relax and open up further. *(Above, left.)*

The water-bladder travels down the vagina and the head of the calf starts to come through the cervix. At this stage the bladder may rupture, though it does not usually do so until the feet of the calf reach the vulva, and by that time the calf's head is through into the anterior vagina. *(Above, right.)*

On an average, this stage is reached after 7 or 8 bouts of second-stage labour strains—usually lasting about half an hour—or a total of between 30 to 40 strains, each strain lasting for from between a half to one second. But with a big calf in a heifer, considerably more time and effort may quite normally be required.

Here you see it as it is inside—head through the cervix and feet at vulva. *(Above.)*

18

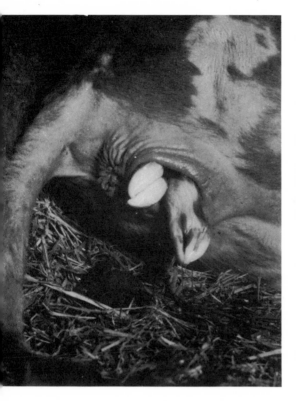

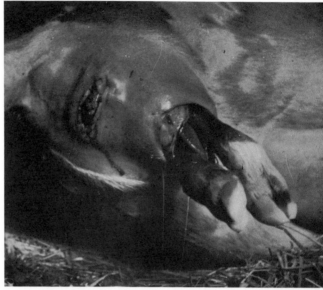

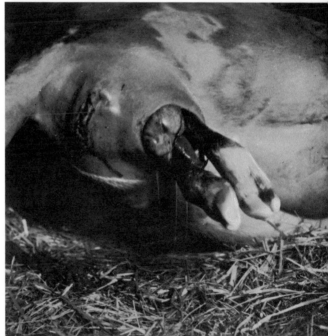

After the appearance of the feet, the intervals between the bouts of straining become shorter, bouts occurring approximately every 15 seconds to 1½ minutes; the number of strains is greater and each one increases in intensity—now lasting from 1 to 2½ seconds. *(Above, left.)*

Thirty to forty of these strains usually sees the calf's tongue appearing. *(Above, right.)* At this stage the patient may rest for a minute or two, to allow the vulva to relax and to gain strength for her final effort. This, again, happens in women.

At least 50 or 60 strains, with varying rest periods of up to 1½ minutes, are now required before the nose of the calf appears. *(Right.)* But again, with Friesian heifers particularly, normal progress may be much slower.

Another 50 will be required before the

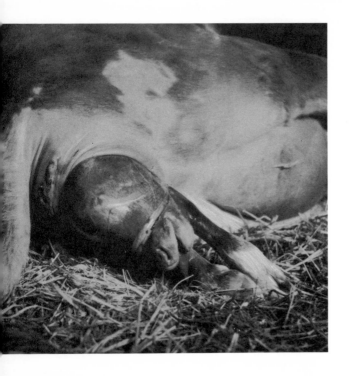

head appears. *(Left.)* During this 50, the rest periods are much shorter—from 15 seconds to 1 minute—and the strains are really intense and prolonged—lasting for up to $2\frac{1}{2}$ seconds—just as though the animal knows that the labour is nearing its completion.

After the head the rest is usually easy—half a dozen intense strains and the calf is half out. *(Below, left.)*

With each strain, as the chest comes through, copious quantities of mucous may pour from the mouth and nostrils. This is a very important point, since it is obviously nature's way of clearing the respiratory passages ready for normal breathing.

Three or four more and the calf is born—alive and unharmed in 999 cases out of 1,000—*provided the mother is left alone.* But more of that later. *(Below, right.)*

In a heifer, this second stage takes on an average between three to six hours, in a cow two to four hours. But with a big calf the second stage may continue quite normally for up to 12 hours or more.

Within two or three minutes, the mother

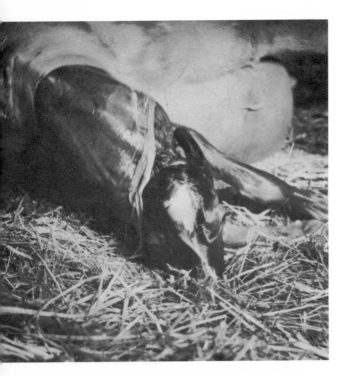

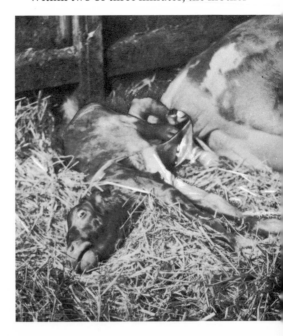

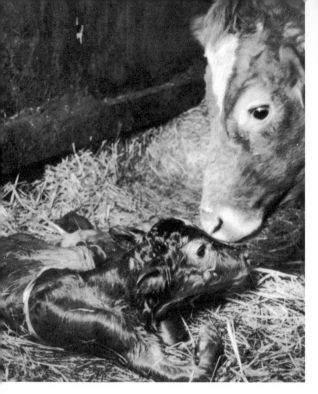

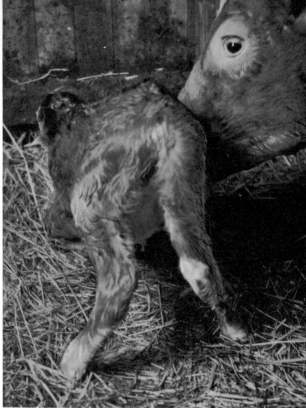

jumps to her feet and starts to lick the calf with a fierce maternal love. *(Above, left.)*

I think all calves should be left to suckle their mothers for at least 48 hours but, of course, on many farms they are taken straight away at birth. I am convinced that leaving the calf with the mother is tremendously advantageous, firstly because the placenta and fluid on the calf contains hormones which play an important part in milk release and subsequent production. And secondly because, during the period between 24 and 36 hours after birth, the calf gets, and can absorb and utilise, all its necessary antibodies against disease contained in the colostrum or first milk of the mother.

The calf is usually staggering onto its legs within 10 or 15 minutes. *(Above, right.)*

Within half an hour, it has found the teats and is sucking down its precious quota of colostrum with its initial laxative and subsequent protective qualities. *(Below.)*

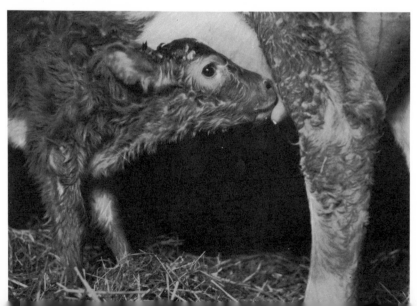

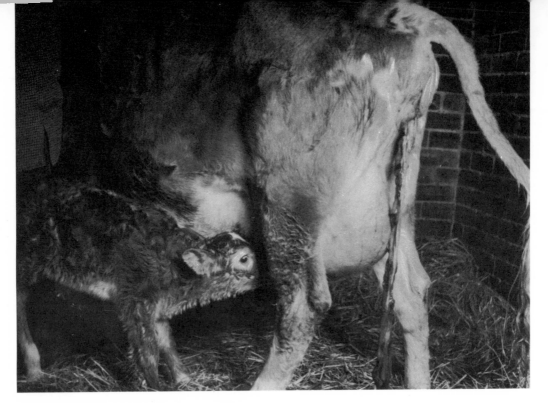

Now comes the third or final stage of the bovine labour—the passing of the afterbirth. *(Above.)* Normally this is passed within an hour or two but occasionally it can hang for several hours. In such cases the retention is usually due to fatigue, perhaps caused by a big calf.

In the heifer photographed, the afterbirth dropped one hour and ten minutes after the calf was born.

Where the afterbirth or cleansing is retained, then special precautions may have to be taken (see Chapter 8 on Afterbirth).

2
Dangers of Premature Interference

AFTER studying the natural birth, it must be obvious just how easy it is to retard nature's progress or to damage a heifer or cow by interfering during labour—during the primary stage of labour, for example, when the cervix is being opened up by the intermittent pressure of the water-bladder.

At this precise stage, the cervical dilation (i.e., the opening up of the womb entrance) is entirely dependent on the water-bladder pressure, especially the pressure exerted on the top part of the cervix. Any manual interference might lead to a premature rupture of the water-bladder and this causes a falling off of

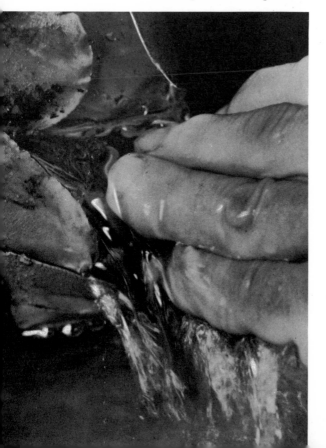

the intra-uterine pressure, the cervix ceases to dilate, and there is a serious set-back to nature's progress. *(Left.)*

I have seen this happen on many occasions, especially in the old days when premature interference was rife.

When the calf is finally presented in the correct position, the cervix is rarely more than three-quarters fully dilated, even though the feet of the calf are now in the passage and the calf's nose may be peeping through. The continuation of the opening up of the cervix is now dependent to a very large extent on the intermittent pressure of the calf's head on the top part of the cervix.

Any interference at this stage will prove disastrous, since roping the feet and pulling forward will jam the calf in the cervix.

This cervix is composed of a powerful ring of muscles and, when the calf is jammed tightly, there occurs a 'spasm' of the muscles—in other words, the relaxation ceases altogether. This means that the

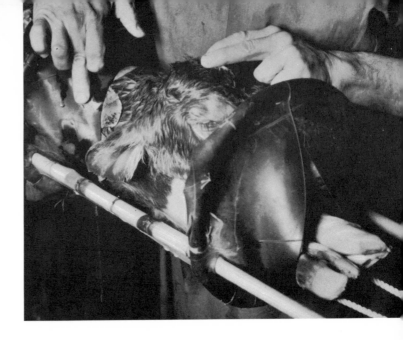

mechanism of natural cervical dilation will no longer function. Further excess traction will rip the cervix and kill the animal. *(Below.)*

In fact, it is certain that manual interference at any time during the passing of the head through the cervix will prove disastrous. I have come across this cervical 'spasm' caused by premature pulling on many, many occasions, and each time it has meant a prolonged embryotomy (i.e. cutting the calf up inside) or, in some cases, a ceasarean section operation.

The next danger period is when the feet of the calf first come into view outside the vulva. In fact, I think this is the most important time of all, because many farmers rope and pull the feet as soon as they appear. *(Above.)*

This is all wrong. When the feet first appear, the cervix may still not be fully dilated, and certainly the vagina and vulva have not had a chance to relax to anything like their full extent. Forced traction or

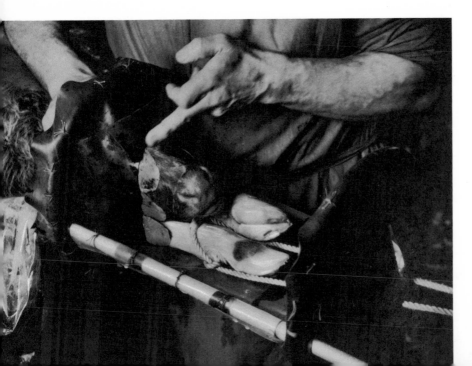

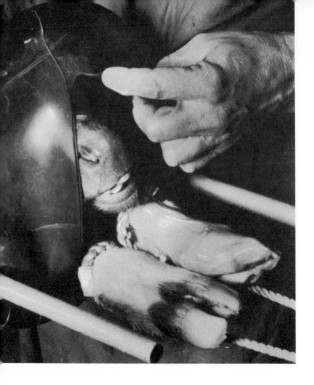

The intermittent straining of labour is designed by nature to maintain the navel supply, but prolonged premature pulling of the calf causes excessively long pressure on the cord and this cuts off the calf's lifeline.

To sum up, therefore, the golden rule with all heifers or cows is to leave the animal to do the job by herself for at least a reasonable period of time, provided that the calf is coming in the correct position and that progress, no matter how slow, continues to be made. (Below.)

When the hind feet of the calf are coming first, i.e. in a posterior presentation, and when the hind feet first appear outside the cow, the cervix is usually only little more

excess pulling at this stage, especially with a big calf, may still cause a ruptured cervix or, at the very least, will produce a torn and lacerated vagina and vulva, with the ever present danger of fatal haemorrhage or secondary sepsis. *(Above.)*

There can be little doubt that the best advice here is that, *provided the calf is straight, and remember only if the calf is straight, leave the animal to complete the birth by herself.* Have patience—the greatest gift of all at calving time. Don't panic so long as progress is being made.

The last thing you should be worrying about is the life of the calf—the calf is much more likely to die if it is pulled away than if it is left to come on its own.

The reason for this is quite simple. Whilst inside the cow, the calf receives its nourishment and oxygen from the mother via the navel cord. It does not start to use its own lungs for breathing until the navel cord ruptures, and this rarely occurs until the calf's head is well outside the cow.

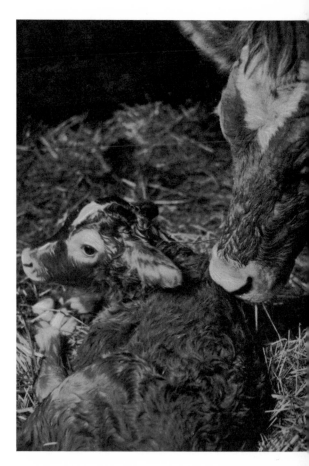

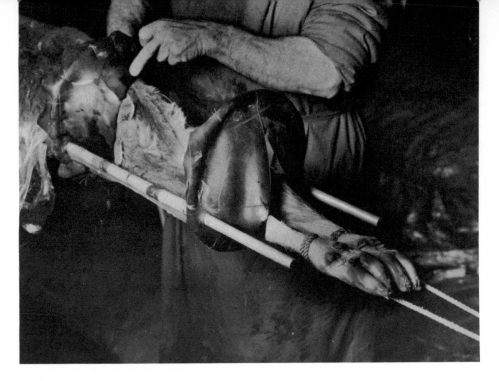

than half open. Excessive pulling on the legs at this stage will nearly always result in a ruptured cervix and a dead animal. The correct technique for dealing with this presentation is dealt with in Chapter 5. *(Above.)*

3
When and How to Examine

OBVIOUSLY it is important to know, with complete confidence, exactly when and how long to leave the patient and when to seek professional advice. The routine measures I advise are these.

If nothing is showing after a period of the intensive straining of second-stage labour—a period of say two hours in a cow and four hours in a heifer—then examine for presentation.

First of all make the time to scrub the hands and arms thoroughly with soap, warm water and antiseptic. *(Below, left.)* It is surprising how few will take the trouble to do this and yet it is of great importance. I've seen many cows die of sepsis as a direct result of examination by a dirty hand.

Now wash the heifer or cow's vulva and perineal region—again a simple precaution often neglected. *(Below, right.)*

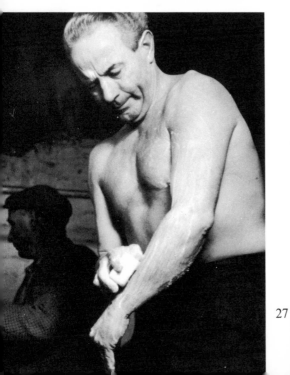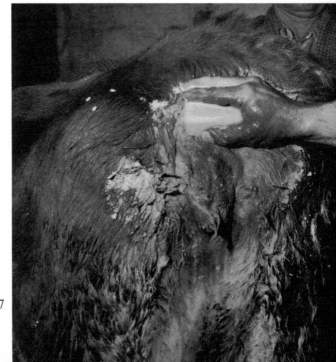

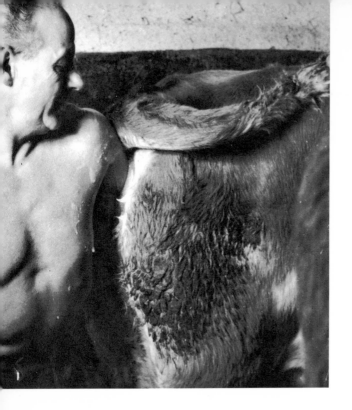

shoulder. If the calf's presentation is wrong, i.e. if the two forefeet and head cannot be felt, then send for the veterinary surgeon at once. *(Left.)*

If the calf's head and forelegs are there, then relax and follow this advice:

If it is spring or summer, turn the animal out with the others and leave her to get on with the job. *(Below, left.)* If it is during the winter, and no loose box is available, accommodate the neighbouring cow elsewhere—this is simple commonsense, because the cow in labour needs some space to stretch out and a neighbour in a double stall is more than likely to tread on her udder. *(Below, right.)*

Tie the patient carefully but loosely with

Insert the hand very slowly and gently, taking great care not to rupture the waterbladder. It is best to strip off for the job because, apart from the fact that it is the only way to be sure of asepsis, you may well have to insert the arm right up to the

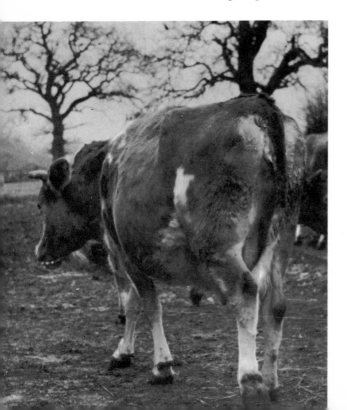

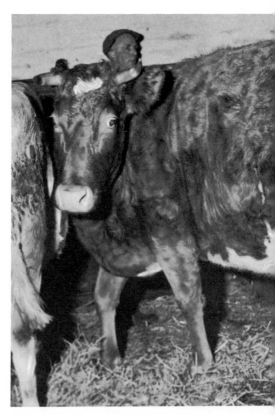

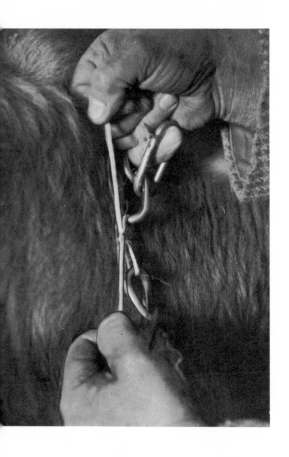

a single link of string in the chain. This is the simple precaution against possible 'hanging' which, I'm glad to say, the majority of herdsmen now adopt instinctively. *(Left.)*

Just one point, though. Never use thick baling string, use a thin strand which is sure to break if the cow hangs back. I've seen several die because the baling string has not broken.

Clear the bedding to one side and cover over the floor with sand or grit. *(Below.)*

This gritting is a very good practical hint, since it is my experience that permanent paralysis after calving is nearly always due to damaged or broken pelvises or hip joints directly caused by slipping about on a greasy floor during labour. *Bedding is not enough—the floor underneath must be completely non-skid.*

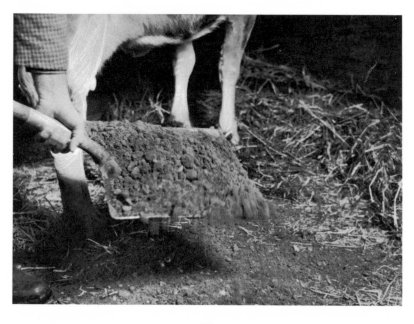

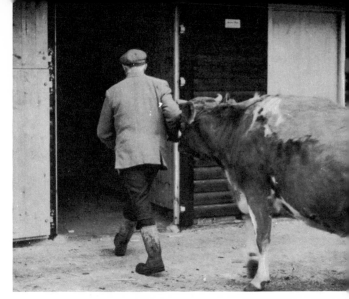

(Above.)

The ideal, however, is to put the patient in a loose box and, again, cover the floor with sand or grit before bedding down. If it is night time, the next thing to do is to go to bed and forget the patient. If it is morning, don't look at her again until late afternoon.

If the floor has not been gritted underneath the bedding, then obturator and/or popliteal paralysis is a common sequel to slipping around during labour. (*Right*).

The obturator and popliteal nerves run down both hind legs and control the muscle and joint movements. Excessive slipping of the leg, usually forward underneath the belly of the cow or heifer, damages these nerves in varying degrees and often results in up to a six-month convalescent period or a trip to the knacker yard.

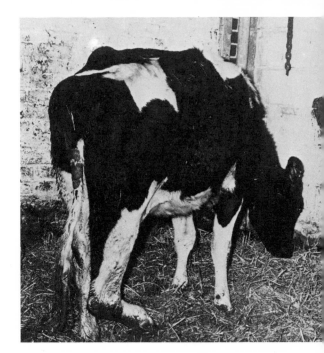

4
General Hints on Assisting

(a) Hobbling and gritting

ONE of the most common, if not the most common, causes of losses in first-calvers is damage to the hips, femurs or pelvis directly caused by slipping and sprawling about on a slippery floor during calving.

Even though the patient is lying comfortably to begin with, she only has to attempt to get up, and in so doing splay her legs once, for irrevocable damage to be done—damage which will mean she will finish up in the knacker's yard.

This is especially the case with the heavier breeds, and I would say that splaying occurs most frequently in Friesian heifers, especially when the calf is by a Friesian bull.

To me these losses are almost criminal, because they can so easily be avoided by following a simple routine.

First of all, clear the bedding from underneath the heifer's hind feet and sprinkle the entire area in front of, between, at the sides and at the back of the legs with sand or grit. *(Right.)* It's *never* enough just to put plenty of bedding down because the restless animal soon pushes the bedding aside. The floor underneath is often as slippery as ice, perhaps because of milk running from the udder.

Now hobble the heifer. Take two short lengths of good strong rope (in an emergency several strands of strong binder twine

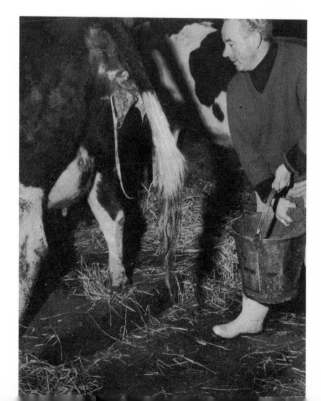

31

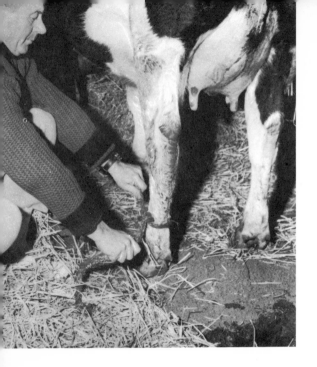

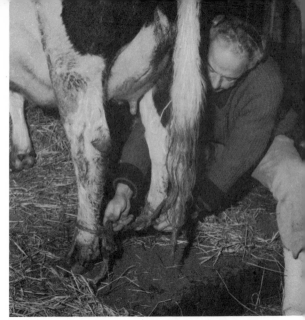

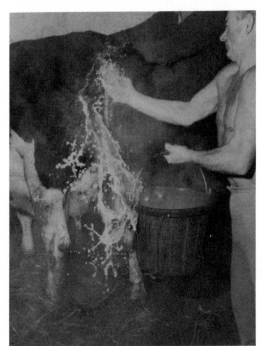

will do), and tie the first length above the heifer's fetlock in a reef knot. *(Above, left.)*

Tie the other piece of rope similarly round the opposite leg and join the two pieces of rope in the centre, again by a tight reef knot. If there are any excessively long loose ends, cut them off with a knife. The right distance apart between the legs—approximately 18 inches—is shown in the picture. *(Above, right.)*

Having fixed the hobble, spread the rest of the sand or grit over as much of the bed area as it will cover.

Now you can get on with the job with all the confidence in the world and the full knowledge that you may have saved your heifer by taking these simple basic precautions. Don't worry about the heifer. She can get up and down with the hobbles fitted and can, if necessary, walk around for days or weeks with them on. *(Right.)*

(b) Lubrication

Many lubricants have been used in bovine obstetrics—liquid paraffin, linseed oil and lard were all favoured by many of the older generation of our profession.

I have found, however, that the best lubricant of all is probably the simplest and most easily obtained—soap flakes. Copious quantities of soap flakes and plenty of hot water produce a lather and lubrication which at times is little short of

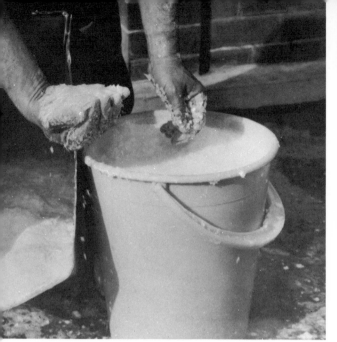

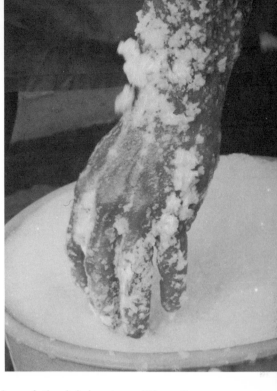

miraculous. *(Above, left.)*

Looking back over twenty-five years of tough practical experience, I can think of many cases where soap flakes have made all the difference between success and failure. I am now so firmly convinced of the value of soap flakes that I buy them by the hundredweight.

I have often heard it said that 'an ounce of lubrication is worth a ton of pressure'. In obstetrics there is much truth in this and I cannot stress too strongly the inestimable value of the lubricant qualities of soap flakes in all cases of difficult or prolonged parturition. *(Above, right.)*

And I would exhort every veterinary student, in particular, to pay great heed to this simple hint. It will prevent many a death and many a frustrating heartache. I only wish someone had told me about soap flakes at the start of my career.

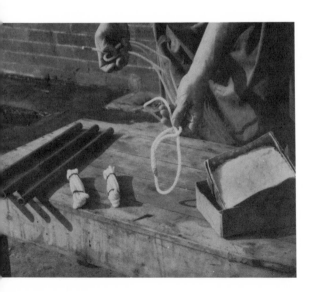

(c) Tools for the job

For the Farmer and Stockman
In addition to the constantly required supply of powerful non-irritant antiseptic, the farmer or stockman should always have in his cupboard or medicine chest: three stout metal bars about two feet long; three nylon calving cords with a fixed noose on one or both ends; and a box of the indispensable soap flakes. *(Left.)*

For the Veterinary Student
In addition to the basic requirements of

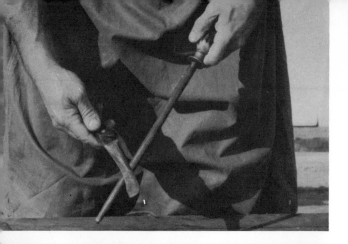

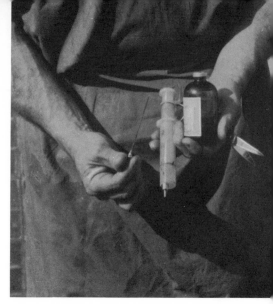

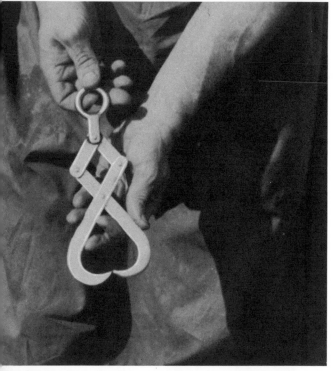

the stockman, the veterinary surgeon should carry first of all a sharp butcher's knife and steel *(above, left)*, not for butchering the cow as so many of my clients have jokingly inferred, but for the simple external embryotomy jobs like amputating the head of the calf or for cutting the foetus in half.

Another extremely valuable instrument for the veterinary surgeon is a self-closing hook which can be used for bringing a head round or fixing any part of the foetus inside the cow. *(Left and below left.)*

Spinal needle, syringe, local anaesthetic and sharp scissors are all vital for the administration of spinal anaesthesia as and when necessary. *(Above, right.)*

Wire cutters, embryotomy wire and flexible wire-tubes are all essential for internal embryotomy, i.e. the cutting up of the foetus inside the cow. *(Below, right.)*

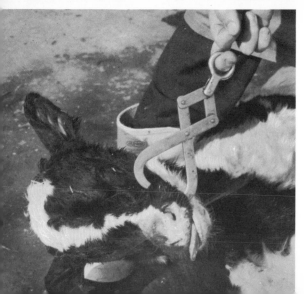

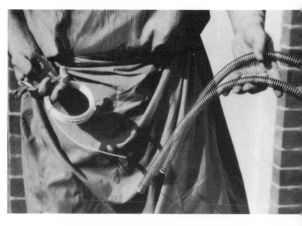

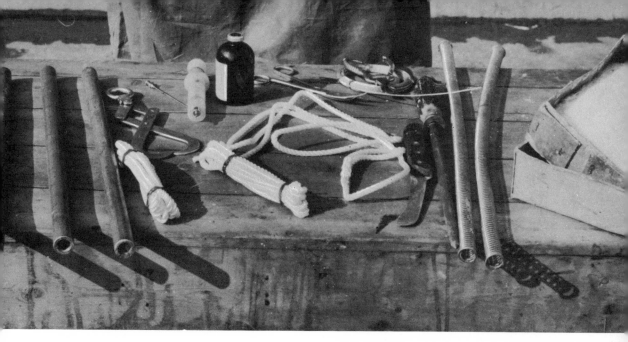

Here then we have the complete calving kit required by any veterinary surgeon to calve any cow. *(Above.)*

You will observe there are no barbaric eye hooks or weird and wonderful instruments. But above all there is no block and tackle, and no so-called calving machine. The skilled, intelligent veterinary surgeon will never use either of these under any circumstances.

(d) Roping a foot and fixing the calving rope to a metal bar

Assistance at calving time should only be given when the animal has ceased to make natural progress. More specific details of when and how to assist are given in later chapters but here, first of all, I illustrate the simple processes of roping a foot, and of fixing the rope correctly to a bar.

These simple hints are important because:

(a) If a calving rope is tied too low down towards the calf's foot, the claw may come off when pulling.

(b) An incorrectly tied knot on the bar is not only liable to slip persistently during the job, but is also often difficult or impossible to untie afterwards. The knot which I illustrate is easily untied, even after the strongest pressure.

Wash the cow's vulva region thoroughly with soap, water and a reliable non-irritant antiseptic, then thoroughly wash your hands and arms. I cannot emphasise too strongly the ever present need for absolute cleanliness during assistance at calving time.

Make a running noose *(Below.)* on the end of a calving rope which has either been

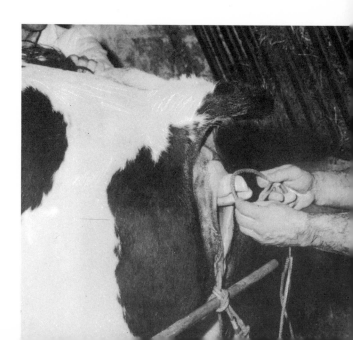

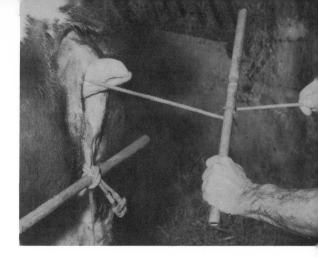

boiled or been soaked in a strong solution of the non-irritant antiseptic.

Fix the noose *above* the calf's fetlock. If the rope is allowed to slip down to the calf's coronet it is liable to come off, pulling the horn of one of the claws with it.

Having fixed the noose, lay the bar on the top side of the rope and pass the end of the rope over and round the bar to form

a half hitch. *(Above.)*

Then take a loop of the free end of the rope forward and pass it underneath the main part, as illustrated. *(Left.)*

Bring the centre of the loop through the larger loop thus formed, by pulling it with

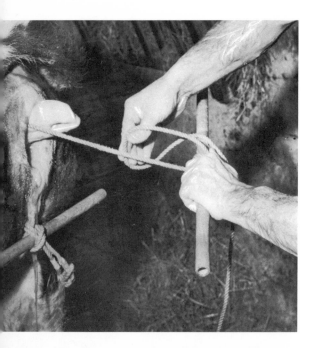

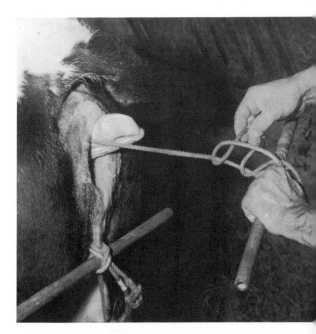

the thumb and forefinger exactly as shown. *(Above.)*

Holding the end of the loop rigidly by the forefinger, pull the bar towards you until the knot tightens. The bar is now fixed by a knot which will stand any amount of pressure but which is comparatively easy to untie. *(Left.)*

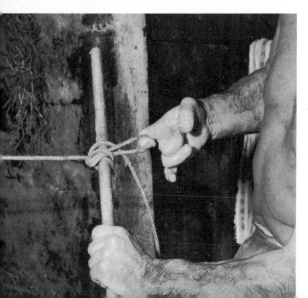

(e) How to assist when the cow or heifer is standing

One of the most difficult tasks is to assist a cow or heifer when she is calving standing up. A heifer, particularly, is often unwilling to lie down during interference—in fact, to get it to lie down, casting is sometimes necessary.

The trouble is that, when pulling by the normal method is tried, it is virtually impossible to exert any effective pressure, and the problem is often complicated by the persistent restless movement of the patient. Here I show an original idea which I have found effective on many occasions.

Having fixed the calving rope to a bar, drape the bar, on both sides of the rope, with a sack or with a towel. *(Right.)*

Now pass one end of the bar underneath the right thigh. *(Below, left.)*

Holding the bar rigidly in position with the right hand, pass the left leg over the other side of the bar. The bar tension can now be taken equally by the backs of both thighs. *(Below, right.)*

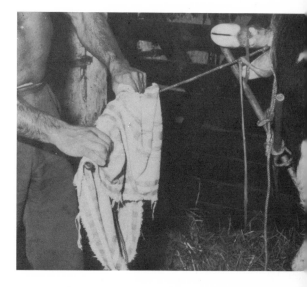

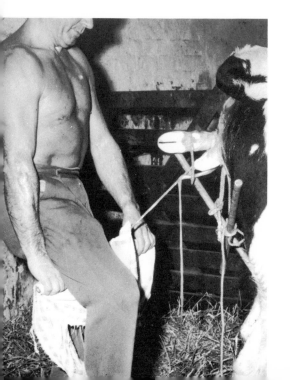

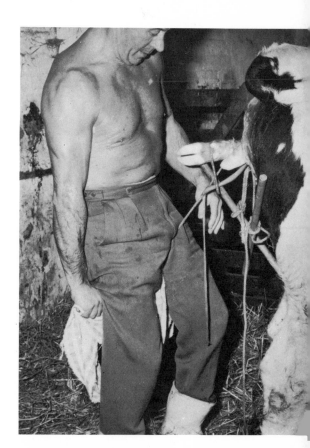

37

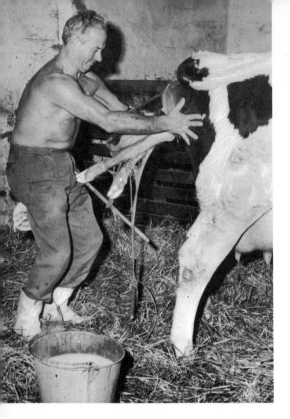

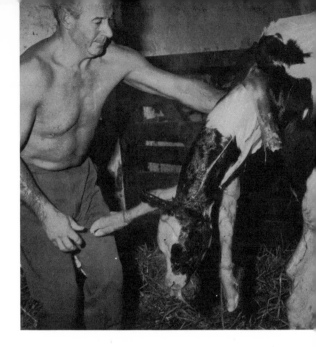

Now place both your hands one on either side of the vulva and, as the cow or heifer strains, push backwards, taking the full weight of the pull on the back of the thighs. The towel or sack helps to cushion the bar and also keeps the trousers reasonably clean. *(Above, left.)*

As progress is made, pressure can be varied in direction by using one arm only and pulling to the one side. *(Above, right.)*

By using this method, at least twice as much power can be obtained as that possible when using the traditional method and, even more important, the fatigue is negligible compared with that associated with arm pulling.

It is very important at all times, whether the heifer is standing or lying, to exert pressure only when the animal strains and to relax completely when the patient relaxes. The old idea of maintaining a steady pressure during assistance is entirely wrong, because steady pressure causes spasm of the uterine neck muscles and holds up the entire process.

(f) Releasing the rope from the bar

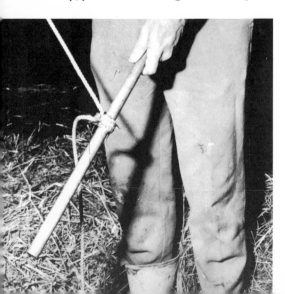

A simple but common problem after assisting a cow or heifer to calve is how to undo the knot on the bar. Even with controlled pulling, the average pair of hefty shoulders can pull the knot remarkably tight. *(Left.)*

With nylon calving ropes costing a fair amount of money, it is important that the rope should not have to be cut, otherwise a new set of ropes will be needed for each calving case. Provided the knot has been tied as illustrated earlier, there is a simple technique for undoing it.

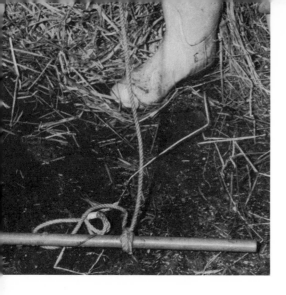

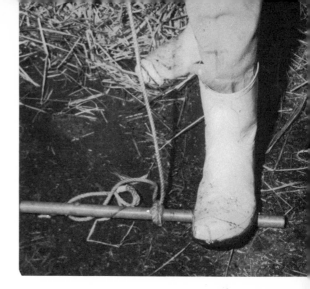

Drop the bar onto the cowshed floor, retaining a hold on the free end of the rope—i.e. the end opposite to the one that has been attached to the calf. *(Above, left.)*

Place the left foot firmly on the bar on one side of the knot. *(Above, right.)*

Bring the right foot onto the other side of the bar and bear all your weight evenly on both feet. Then wrap the free end of the rope several times round the hand. *(Below, left.)*

If the knot is very tight, it's a good idea to protect the hand with a towel or piece of sacking before wrapping the rope around. Using two hands, pull with all your strength. A tight knot will require considerable upward pulling, but I have yet to see one which did not untie by this method. *(Below, right.)*

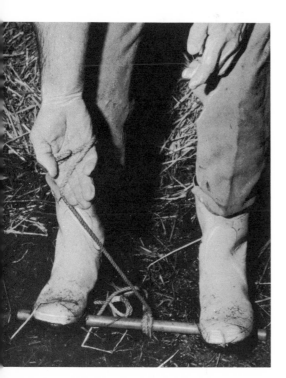

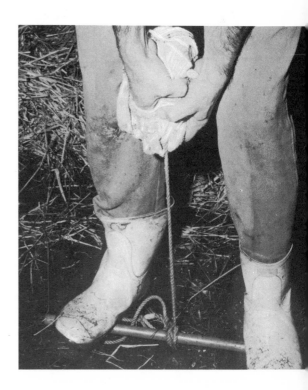

(g) Deficiency delay

Often I am called out to attend cows coming down with their third or fourth calf. The history usually is that they have been shaping for calving for anything up to sixteen hours but are not getting on with the job.

In such cases the trouble, almost invariably, is caused by calcium deficiency.

It is very important to know about this 'deficiency delay' because any attempt to pull the calf away from such patients can, and often does, result in a prolapsed womb and a dead cow.

The first step is to see how the calf lies. Having scrubbed up and lubricated thoroughly, insert the hand very carefully, taking great care not to rupture the water bladder. Examine for the calf's two fore feet and head. If they are there, then the calf is straight and properly presented and the cow will most assuredly calve it. *(Right and below.)*

This examination in 'delay' cases is really a job for your veterinary surgeon and one you shouldn't tackle unless you are very experienced and quite unable to get professional help. The reason this examination is so much trickier than in

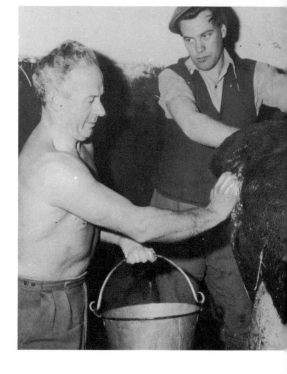

straightforward labour is that usually the calf is right inside the womb and the cervix may only be partially dilated.

Once it is established that the calf is presented correctly, you may be almost sure that all that is needed is 16 oz of calcium boro-gluconate solution. The calcium should be injected underneath the

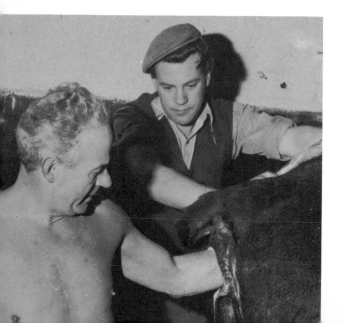

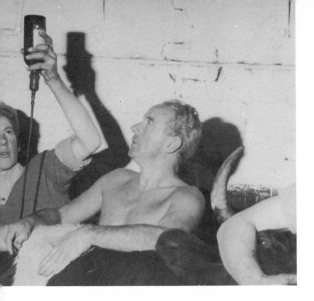

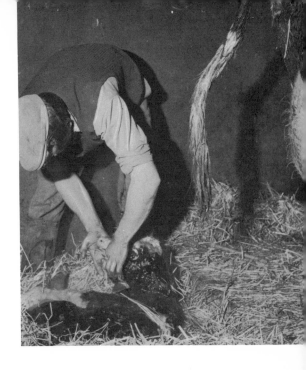

skin, approximately a handsbreadth behind the central ridge of the scapula (main
bone of the shoulder joint). *(Above.)*

The correct technique is not so easy as it
looks and this is another reason why the
treatment should be given only by a
veterinary surgeon.

Another essential feature of the calcium
injection—a thorough 'rubbing away' of
the injection swelling. This is essential not
only to ensure rapid absorption of the
solution, but also to avoid abscesses and
permanently unsightly lumps. *(Below.)*

Calcium injected subcutaneously takes
approximately twenty minutes to take

effect. At the end of that time the cow
will go into normal powerful second-
stage labour and will deliver the calf by
herself. *(Above.)*

*In all such cases of protracted labour, the
cow should be left to calve herself after the
calcium administration. Calcium deficiency
causes a loss of muscular control in the neck
of the uterus (womb) and, consequently, if
the calf is 'pulled out', there is great danger
that the womb will prolapse behind it.*

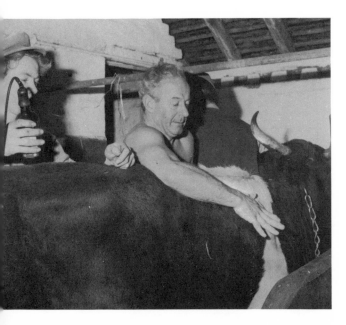

5
When and How to Assist

THE COW or heifer has been examined—the calf has been found to be presented correctly (i.e. two fore-feet and head coming)—and the patient has either been put in a 'non-skid' loose box or has been tied with string on a gritted shippon floor. The next obvious question is just how long such cases can be safely left before doing something about it?

It is difficult to generalise but, provided the foetus is presented correctly (and I cannot stress this point too often), the patients can be left with complete safety for a further eight to twelve hours. (Below.)

In other words, if the calving is not completed by the following morning (if you have left the patient over-night) or by late afternoon (if the examination was done in the morning), then the veterinary surgeon should be called in. He will decide whether to assist or whether to leave her to her own devices for a further period, depending on the size of the calf, progress being made, and the general state of cervical, vaginal, and vulval relaxation.

However, there are occasions when a keen practical farmer or stockman can detect the cessation of progress in the birth and can intelligently assist by

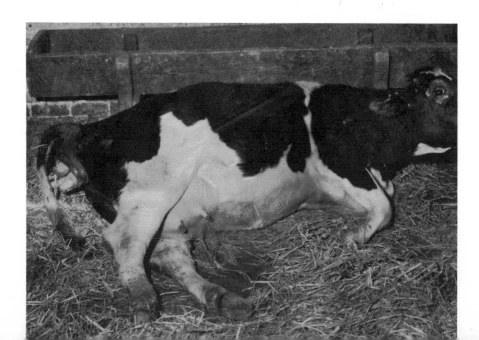

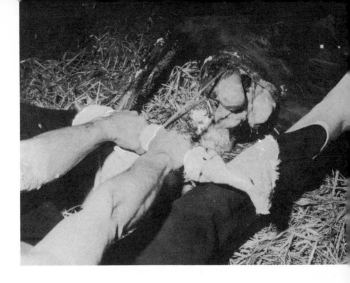

himself, or at least attempt to do so, before consulting his veterinary surgeon, or perhaps more important, know how to assist if the veterinary surgeon is not immediately available. I am thinking particularly of three fairly common situations—when the calf's nose has been showing for some time and the head and tongue are swelling markedly; when the calf is apparently 'stuck at the hips'; and when the hind feet are coming first.

Before dealing with these, however, I want to emphasise probably the most important point of all in the calving of heifers or cows.

Excess force should never be used. In the vast majority of cases no more than one man, and one man only, should be allowed to pull on the ropes, and then only when the animal strains. In the few instances where two people are allowed to pull, they must do so only under strict veterinary supervision. I have proved many times that, in the odd cases where nature fails (and provided you wait until natural progress ceases), one man with soap flakes lubrication and lots of patience can calve the tightest and most difficult case. (Above.)

The only time any form of excess traction is permissible is when the calf is dead and putrified, because then the rotten calf will stretch or give before the cervix will tear or the vagina and vulva rupture.

(a) Nose presented with head and tongue swollen

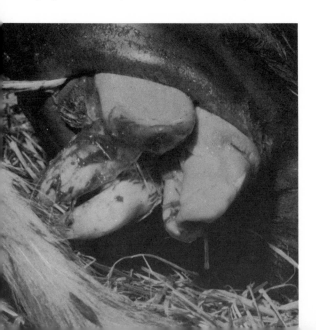

In a heifer, when the nose of the calf has been showing for three hours or longer and no further progress has been made, then assistance is required because, after that length of time in such a position, the calf's head and tongue may become markedly swollen. *(Left.)*

The tendency in such cases is to rely entirely on pulling on the feet of the calf. Although it is often necessary to pull on the legs alternately, this in itself does not usually work, because it merely tends to bring both shoulders forward and increase the impaction. I have found the best procedure to be as follows:

43

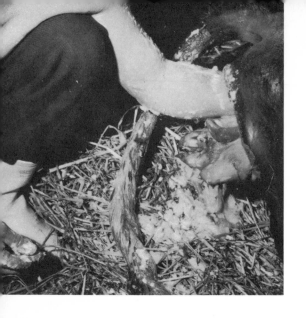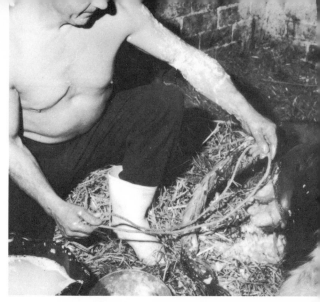

Having first sanded or gritted the floor underneath the bedding and hobbled the heifer as described in a previous chapter, thoroughly wash the hands and arms as well as the heifer's vulva and perineal region. Then take several handfuls of soap flakes and with them and the hot water lubricate between the top of the calf's head and the top of the vagina. *(Above, left.)*

Next, take one of the nylon calving ropes which has either been boiled or soaked in a strong solution of non-irritant antiseptic and make it into a loop. *(Above, right.)*

Insert the centre part of the loop over the top of the calf's head to just behind the ears *(below)*, keeping the free ends of the rope outside the vulva. *(Right.)*

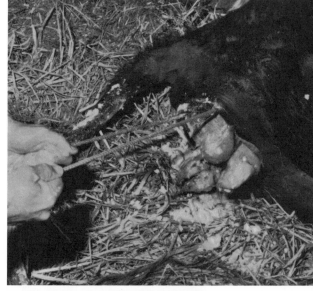

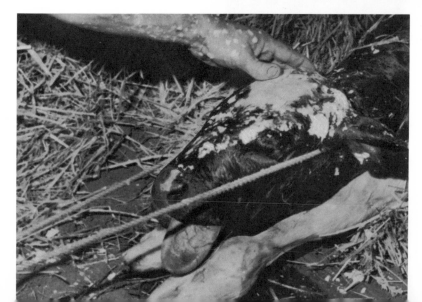

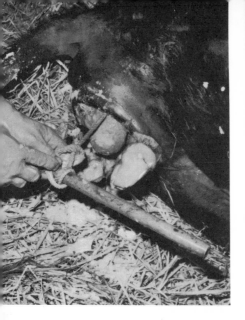
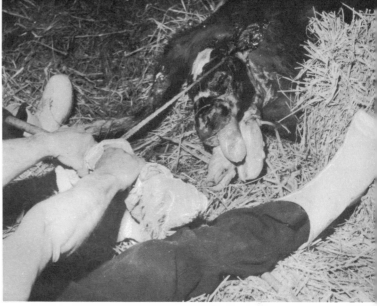

Tie the ends to a bar and then, as the heifer strains (and only as the heifer strains), moderate pressure on the bar will soon bring the head forward. *(Above, left and right.)*

It will probably be necessary to rope and bar both the forelegs, and to pull on these in turn with the head rope, before the head finally emerges from the vulva. Once the head of the foetus is delivered, the rest of the job is usually easy.

During the assistance, a solid bale of straw placed between the heifer's hind end and one foot not only prevents the heifer moving backwards, but considerably helps the effectiveness of the pulling.

(b) Stuck at the hips

(Left.)

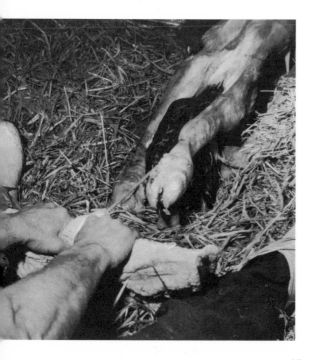

The next presentation where interference is necessary is where the foetus apparently gets 'stuck at the hips'. This occurs fairly commonly, especially in Friesian heifers.

In such cases there is always the feeling that a little more help is all that is required and the farmer often seeks additional help, finishing up pulling the heifer round and round the box and sometimes even round the outside yard. *Never be tempted to do this, or for that matter to employ any form of excess strength, because force is completely contra-indicated and will most assuredly kill or permanently damage the mother, besides inflicting a great deal of unnecessary pain.*

It is likely the case may be one for the veterinary surgeon but there are several emergency first-aid methods which should always be tried before sending for him.

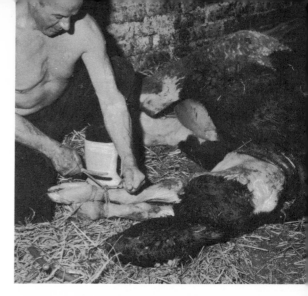

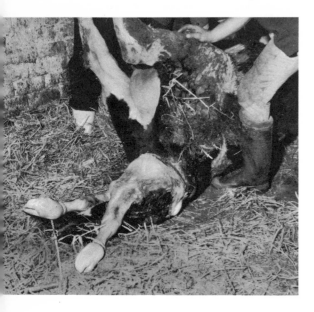

(Above.)

First of all, turn the heifer or cow onto her back, then over onto the side opposite to the one you found her on. Leave her completely alone for five minutes, then try the gentle assistance of one person as and when she strains. This simple procedure, and nothing else, will release fifty per cent of the calves in such cases.

If this fails, rope the forelegs of the foetus together using a figure of eight knot. Tie the knot as tight as possible. *(Top, right.)*

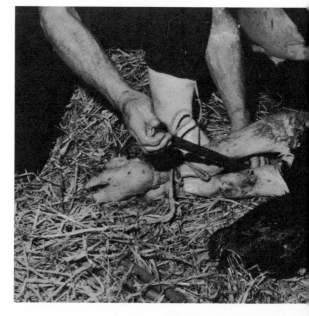

Insert a bar between the tied legs and slip the bar up to the calf's elbows. *(Centre, right.)*

With someone pulling on the ropes, and again only as the patient strains, rotate the foetus on its own axis—first in one direction and then in the other. This will release most of the other cases. *(Bottom, right.)*

Two other tips might be tried.

First of all, pass a strong sack under-

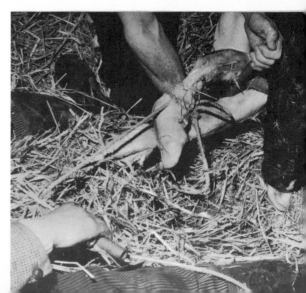

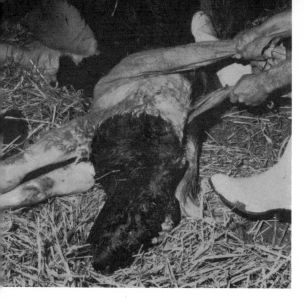

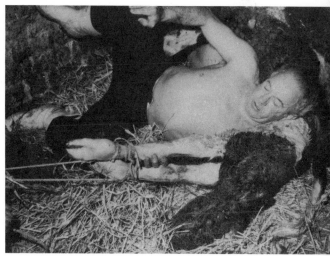

(Below.)
opposite direction. In this case it is worth trying to twist the foetus simultaneously, first in one direction and then in the other.

If all these methods fail, send for your veterinary surgeon. He will probably cut the calf away in the manner described in the following section on Embryotomy.

neath the body of the calf and as close to the vulva as possible. Gripping both ends of the sack firmly, pull as strongly as possible at right angles to the long axis of the mother. At the same time, get the assistant to pull downwards on the legs. The idea here is to assist the stifles of the foetus over the brim of the mother's pelvis and I have used this successfully on a number of occasions. *(Above.)*

Alternately, and based on the same principle, push one shoulder underneath the diaphram of the calf and lever outwards as the assistant pulls downward in the

(c) Embryotomy

Embryotomy simply means the cutting up of a foetus while the foetus is still inside the cow, whether the foetus is lying wholly or partially in the uterus.

This, of course, is a job for a veterinary surgeon but a knowledge of the method employed is not only interesting, but it should assist agricultural students and farmers to understand better the tasks of the veterinary surgeon. It should also highlight the tremendous advantages of embryotomy over forced traction.

It must be said, however, that this section is applicable chiefly to the veterinary reader.

When animals are interfered with prematurely, a spasm of the cervical muscles occurs, and the foetus jams in an incompletely opened cervix. When this happens, embryotomy is not only essential but it becomes arduous and complicated—legs have to be peeled off, the body of the foetus has to be whittled down in size, etc, etc.

However, by allowing the animal to progress naturally, the need for extensive complicated embryotomy disappears completely. In fact, if nature is given a reasonable chance, embryotomy is required only for the following:

1. Amputation of a turned-back head

when the foetus is emphysehatous (i.e. when it is dead and blowing up with putrefying gases).

2. Very occasionally in a breach presentation (i.e. when the calf's tail is coming

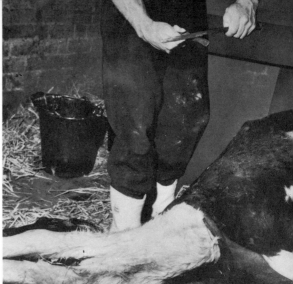

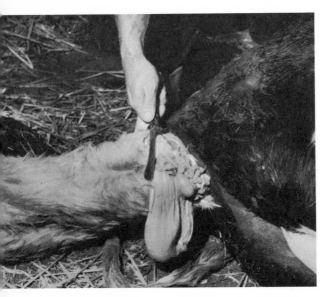

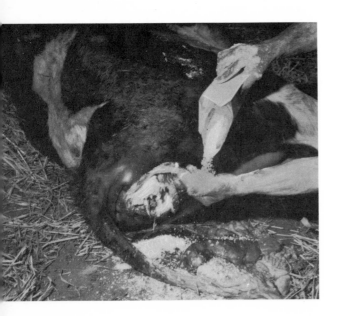

first), when the leg joints are stiffened (ankylosed) and it is not possible to bend the hock forward or the fetlock backward.

3. When the foetus gets stuck with the hips in the pelvis of the mother.

4. In a 'schistosoma reflexus' (i.e. a monstrosity where the foetus is turned inside out), when the rudimentary legs are pointing downwards into the uterus. When the rudimentary legs are presented, especially in a heifer, then a caesarean section is usually indicated.

Undoubtedly the commonest of these four indications is No. 3, i.e. when a dead foetus is stuck at the hips and all the rational efforts described in the previous chapter have failed to move it. The embryotomy technique is as follows.

First of all, using a sharp butcher's knife, cut the foetus in half as close to the patient's vulva as possible. (A spinal anaesthetic may have to be administered, depending on the duration of the labour and degree of exhaustion of the patient). *(Above and top, left.)*

Next, cover the stump with a copious quantity of sulpha powder. This is a simple precaution but well worth using as a routine. The sulpha drug helps to control any infection over and around the vulva area. *(Bottom, left.)*

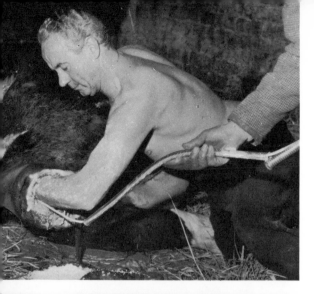

Thread a calving rope through one of the flexible wire tubes, and pass the looped end of the calving rope into the uterus and over the top of the tail of the foetus. *(Top, left.)*

Pass the hand around the hind end of the foetus to between the two stifle joints. Feel for the cord loop and, when you find it, pull it to just outside the vulva—having simultaneously guided the metal spring along the vagina to the foetal tail region to protect the delicate tissues of the mother from the rough surface of the wire. *(Centre, left.)*

Tie a good length of embryotomy wire to the loop. A well tied reef knot is essential here, even though the wire is not easy to handle. *(Bottom, left.)*

Thread the wire through the second wire tube. It is usually necessary to use a second calving cord to do this—i.e. pass the cord through the spring, tie the other end of the wire to the loop of the cord, and then pull it through. *(Below.)*

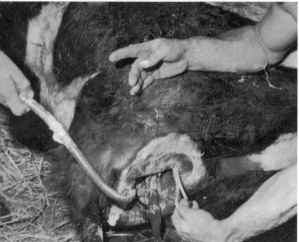

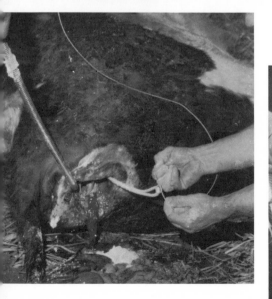

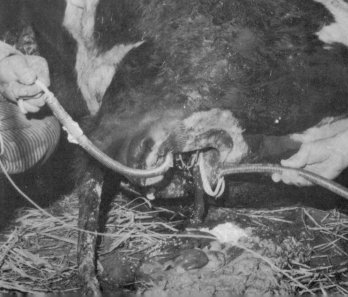

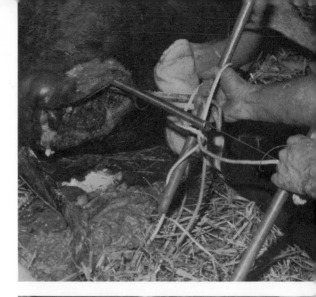

Cup the hand over the junction of the wire and cord and, as the assistant pulls the cord through the first metal spring, guide the second spring into the position between the thighs of the foetus. Tie each end of the wire to a bar, cross the springs over each other, and start to saw. *(Top, right.)*

It takes only a few seconds to saw through the pelvis of the foetus and the hind quarters can then be easily removed in two halves. *(Bottom, right.)* The mother is completely undamaged and, within minutes of the operation, will sit up and start to eat or drink.

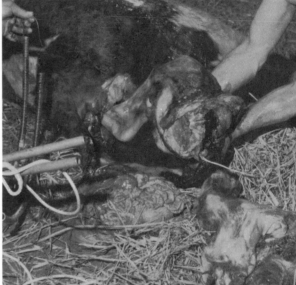

The tremendous advantage of this simple embryotomy over the forced extraction by calving implements, gangs of men, a block and tackle or tractor is self evident and crystal clear. The illustration of this fact is probably my main reason for including this section on embryotomy.

Exactly the same technique is used for the amputation of the head of the foetus, the cutting off of an ankylosed hind leg, and the amputation of portions of the schiztosoma. In each case the job can be done quickly and efficiently, without any damage whatsoever to the mother.

(d) Posterior presentation

When a calf is being born hind feet first, the common idea is that it suffocates by breathing in the fluids from the uterus (or womb). This is not so, at least not until the calf is nearly born, because so long as the navel cord remains intact, the calf is kept alive by blood which flows in through the cord from the mother.

The calf does not use its own lungs for breathing until the navel cord ruptures, and this does not occur until the calf is nearly born—*certainly not before the entire hind end of the calf is outside the vulva.*

The following series of pictures will show how to get a *live* calf in a posterior presentation and, if the instructions are followed carefully, a dead calf in these circumstances will be a comparative rarity.

Usually when the calf is coming backwards, the cow takes longer than normal to get the feet out and she doesn't appear to strain anything like as hard as when the calf's fore feet and head are presented correctly. This is because, in the posterior

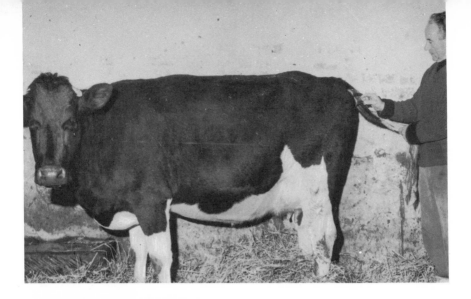

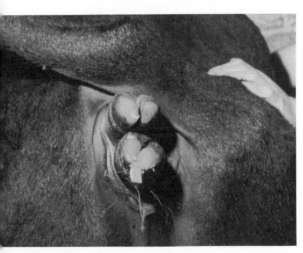

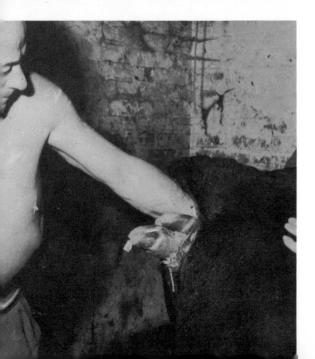

presentation, there is no head to exert pressure on the top part of the cervix after the rupture of the water bladder. (*Above.*)

How to tell when the calf is coming hind feet first? Simply by the fact that the claws, or feet, are upside down. It is surprising how often some stockmen forget this elementary rule of diagnosis. (*Centre, left.*)

Nonetheless, it is wise to make sure that they are hind feet, because the calf may be coming upside down. Scrub up thoroughly and examine for the hocks and tail. (*Bottom, left.*)

At this stage there is no need to panic. In fact, it is quite safe and often wise to allow the cow or heifer two, three or even four hours of normal straining after the hind feet appear.

This gives the cervix (or neck of the womb) time to relax and open up completely. Because there is no head to exert pressure on the top part of the cervix, the womb takes longer to open. Consequently, premature pulling can be disastrous, as illustrated on the model in a previous chapter.

A veterinary surgeon called in the early stages of a posterior presentation will often inject a muscle relaxant intravenously and leave the patient for an hour or so before proceeding to help. Obviously, therefore, it is much better to have a veterinary surgeon supervise the birth.

Having confirmed that they are hind legs, and having waited until the cervix

51

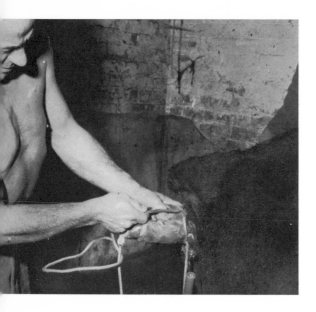

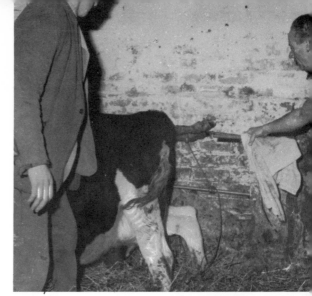

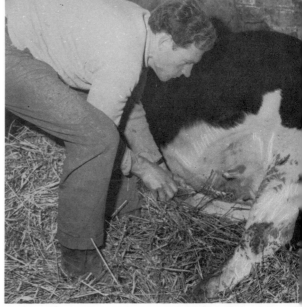

is opened up, rope both feet above the fetlocks and fix the ropes to bars as instructed previously. *(Above.)*

One person, and only one person should pull on the bars, pulling one leg at a time and only when the animal strains.

Even with only one pulling, when pressure is applied the patient will often go down. When this happens, release the pressure immediately so that the cow will not sprawl awkwardly. If the patient is a heifer, of course, the legs will be hobbled and sprawling will be a lot less likely. *(Top, right.)*

If and when the cow does go down, always make her comfortable by pulling both her hind legs out from underneath her. Needless to say, the job of assisting is very much easier with the cow lying down. *(Centre, right.)*

When the calf's hocks appear outside the cow's vulva, it usually means that the entire hind end of the calf has passed through the cow's pelvis and cervix and is now in the vagina (or passage). When this stage is reached, the rest of the job is usually comparatively easy. *(Bottom, right.)*

Often when the calf's hind end comes

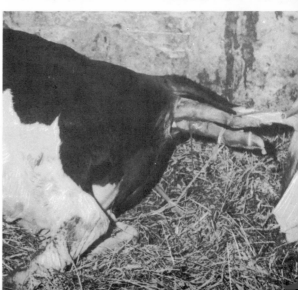

52

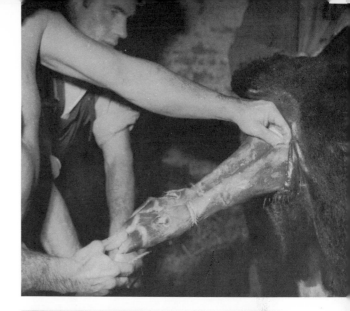

into the passage the cow will get to her feet or attempt to do so. It is wise to allow her to stand and relax for a few minutes if she wishes to do so. Almost invariably, when further assistance is attempted, she will lie down on her opposite side.

This is nature's way of helping delivery by changing the area of abdominal pressure on the calf. (*Top, right.*)

At this stage, the pulling should still be confined to one person, persisting on one leg at a time and only as the cow strains. The reason why it is essential to maintain this intermittent pulling is that blood must be allowed to flow freely through the navel cord, otherwise the calf will certainly die. When the cow strains, the flow is interrupted for a few seconds by the pressure on the cord between the cow's pelvis and the calf's abdomen or chest. But, when the cow relaxes between each strain, the precious blood supply is resumed. (Below.)

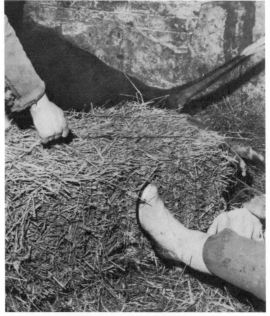

The old traditional idea of 'maintaining a steady pull' is absolutely wrong and has been responsible for the loss of countless calves. The 'steady pull' idea should be banished from stockmens' minds now and for ever.

When the patient is down, a useful hint is to place a bale of straw between her hind end and the feet of the assistant. This allows the single-handed puller to exert much more effective pressure during the cow's strains. (*Right.*)

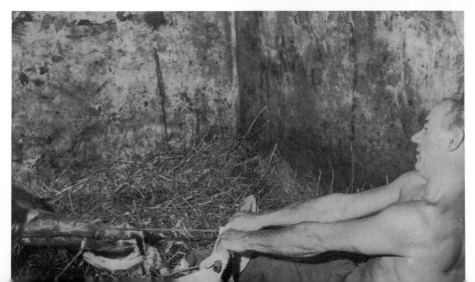

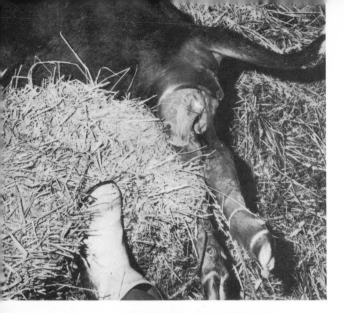

end of the calf is outside the vulva it is a matter of urgency that the calf should be got out quickly. *(Top, left.)*

At this stage, the navel cord is trapped tightly between the cow's pelvis and the lower part of the calf's chest, and the life-giving blood supply from the mother is cut off. And the cord may rupture at any moment—when that happens, the calf will involuntarily breathe in and fill its lungs with the uterine fluids.

Consequently, as soon as the hind end of the calf is out, get several men to help and pull like hell. You have approximately 30 to 40 seconds in which to get a live calf. You won't injure the cow at this stage, because the widest part of the calf's chest is now through the mother's pelvis and cervix. *(Centre, left.)*

Where the calf is alive when assistance is started, it will have a ninety-nine per cent chance of survival if this routine is adhered to. *(Below.)*

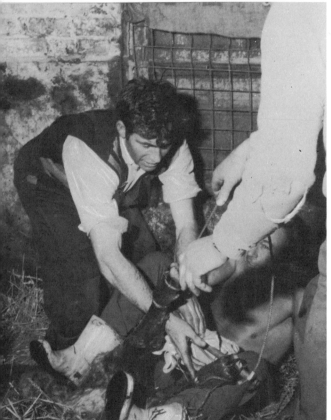

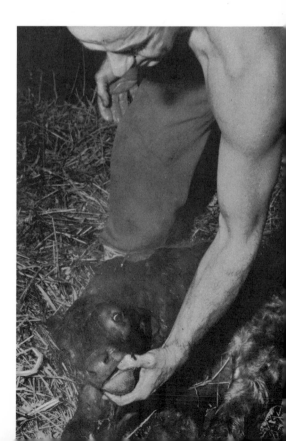

Up to the present assistance should be casual, calm, and completely unhurried. But, and this is the most important point of the whole series, as soon as the entire hind

6
How to Resuscitate a Calf

MANY calves' lives are lost through lack of a simple knowledge of the means of inducing the all-important first gasp of breathing.

Such loss of life occurs chiefly when the calf is born backwards, due to the fact that the navel cord ruptures while the head and chest of the calf are still inside the cow. Rupture of the cord usually occurs as soon as the entire hind end of the calf is outside the cow's vulva.

In practically every case when the calf appears to be dead, the heart is still beating. If you succeed in inducing a single gasp of air into the lungs, the calf can often be saved.

There are four simple methods of producing that breathing reflex.

Straw in the Nose *(Right.)*
Insert a fairly rigid piece of straw into the calf's nostril and push up as far as you like. Continue to move the straw up and down inside the nostril for about five or six seconds. In many cases, the calf will shake its head and start to breathe.

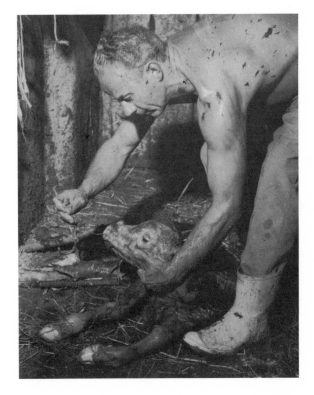

'The Kiss of Life'

If the straw fails to produce a reflex, open the calf's mouth, hold the tongue forward on the floor of the mouth with one hand, and blow down the calf's throat.

In this, all you are doing is blowing carbon dioxide into the calf's respiratory system—carbon dioxide is a well known and very valuable respiratory stimulant. Continue blowing down for at least a minute. *(Right.)*

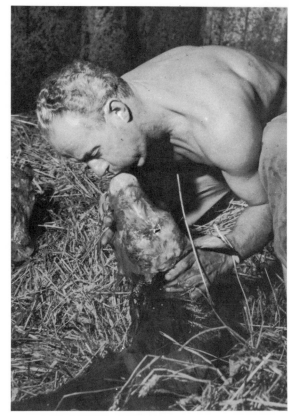

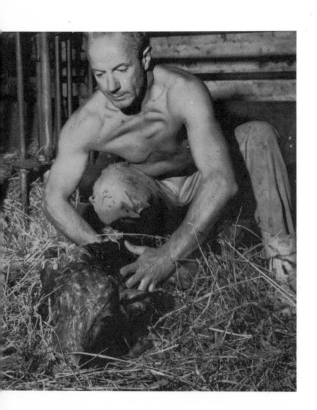

Artificial Respiration

Artificial respiration is of tremendous value in a calf and can be continued for five or ten minutes. *(Left.)*

The calf should be placed on its brisket, with its forelegs stretched out in front and its head resting on them. Intermittent pressure should be applied with the palms of the hands over the back portion of the chest cavity. The best way to judge the correct position here is to try to have the back of the palm over the diaphragm.

When using artificial respiration, it is a good idea to have an assistant administering the 'Kiss of Life' at intervals of about twenty seconds.

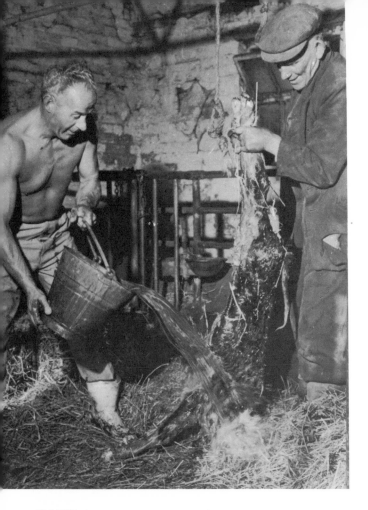

Cold Water

Get an assistant to hold the calf upside down, or suspend the calf down by means of a rope tied over a beam, and throw a bucket of cold water over the chest and head regions. This may seem a bit drastic, but I have found it successful when the straw and carbon dioxide have failed.

7
Simple Malpresentations

ONLY a qualified veterinary surgeon should attempt to correct a malpresentation. Even a comparatively inexperienced qualified assistant in a country veterinary practice has had more experience of malpresentations than the average farmer or herdsman.

This is simply because trouble at calving time on the individual farm is comparatively uncommon whereas, in a veterinary practice, trouble is our business. In fact, the average veterinary surgeon rarely sees a normal calving.

However, the veterinary surgeon is not always immediately available and, if the malpresentation is a simple one, then an intelligent herdsman should be able to cope in an emergency. In any case, the techniques described in this section should be of great interest to all stockmen and farmers and should prove of considerable value to veterinary students.

(a) Head turned right back

This is a common malpresentation and, although its correction is comparatively easy in a cow, in a heifer the job can be extremely difficult.

If the cow is in a loose box, secure its head and tie it up with a halter. This precaution may seem elementary but it's surprising how often examination and assistance is attempted with the patient continually moving around.

A first essential at all calving cases, before any form of examination or interference is attempted, is an abundance of hot water and plenty of powerful though non-irritant antiseptic. *(Right.)*

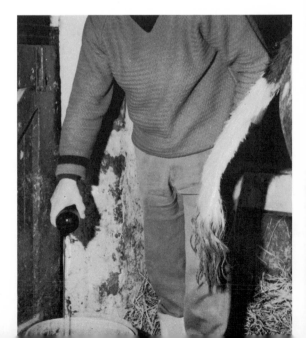

58

As suggested earlier, it is much better to strip off for all calving cases. It is the only way that complete cleanliness can be attained, and it allows one to insert the arm up over the shoulder joint. Having thoroughly washed the cow's vulva and the hand and arm, examine for presenta- *(Below.)*

It is necessary to get right inside to assess the calf's position. In the case illustrated, the calf's head was turned sharply back along the left-hand side of the uterus. *(Below.)*

To set about rectifying such a presentation, first of all place the flat of the hand on the calf's brisket and push it back into the uterus in the intervals between the cow's strains. *(Centre, right.)*

This illustrates exactly what's being done inside at this stage. *(Bottom, right.)*

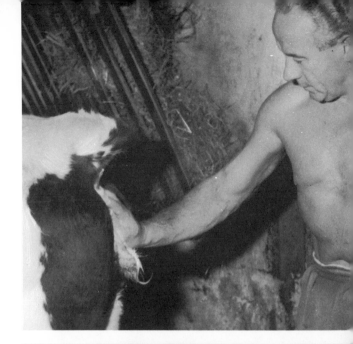

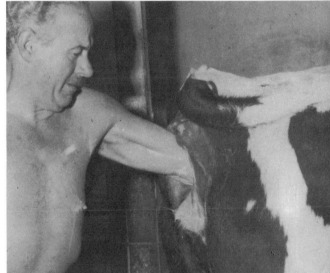

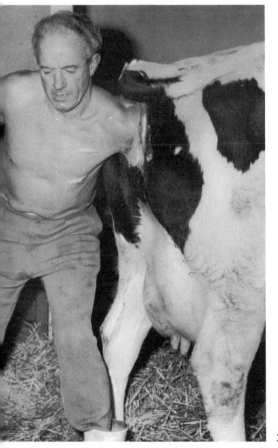

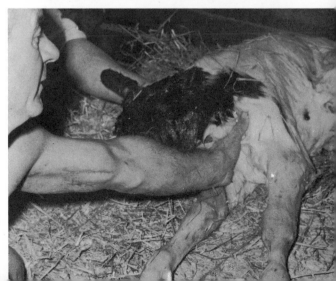

59

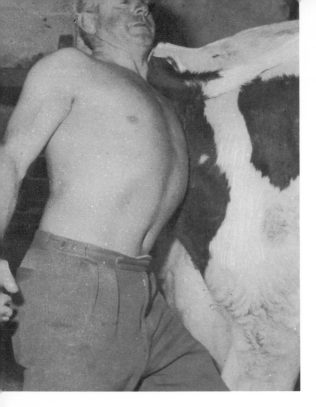

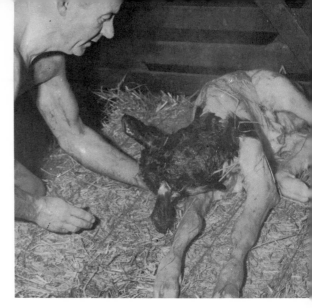

With the calf completely back in the uterus, pass the left hand (or right hand if you happen to be right handed) along from the calf's ear to underneath the jaw. *(Above, left and right.)*

Turn your body away from the cow so that your back is facing the cow's head and, in this position, lever the calf's head round. Of course, you have to be fit and fairly strong for this job, but most veterinary surgeons are. *(Below, left.)*

This shows exactly what is being done inside the cow in the previous illustration. *(Below, right.)*

In the vast majority of cases in cows, as soon as the head is straightened, the calf will be pushed out rapidly. However, in heifers, it is often possible only partially to straighten the head, owing to the lack of sufficient room. This causes an S-shaped bend which is dealt with in the next section.

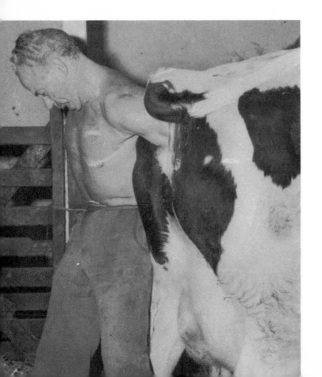

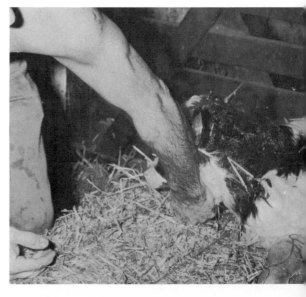

(b) S-bend hold up

Often in a heifer, and occasionally in a cow where the calf is very large, it is difficult or impossible to straighten out by hand a head which has turned right back.

What happens is that, although one can bring the calf's nose round to the entrance of the cervix or opening of the womb (i.e. so that it rests on the cow's pelvis), there is an S-shaped bend in the calf's neck. Each time the cow strains, or if pressure is exerted on the calf's feet, the head stays where it is or twists back again.

There is a simple method of overcoming this.

First of all, take a calving rope which has either been boiled or soaked for several minutes in a strong solution of non-irritant antiseptic. *(Top, right.)*

Having thoroughly washed and lubricated the vulva and the hands and arms, insert the loop of rope into the vagina. *(Below.)*

Pass it along over the top of the calf's head to just behind the ears, maintaining a moderate pressure with your other hand on both of the free ends of the rope all the while. *(Bottom, right.)* You will find this is necessary because, inside, you have to put the loop over one ear at a time and, unless

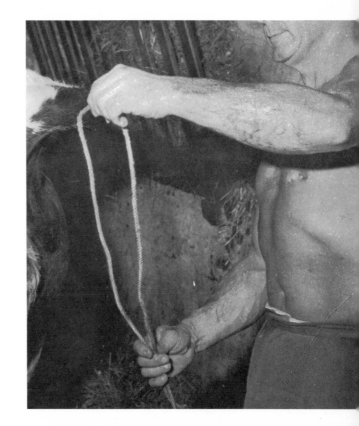

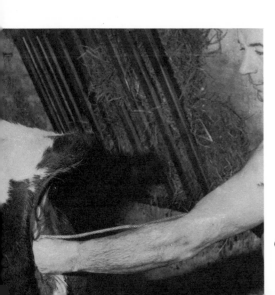

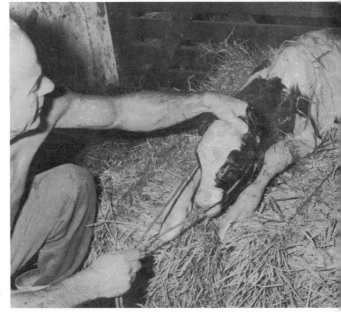

61

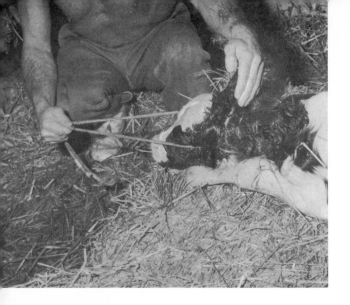

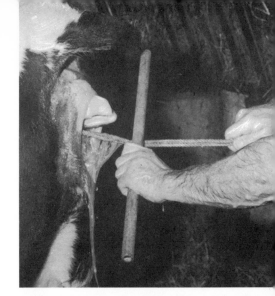

a steady pressure is maintained, the loop slips off the first ear as you are adjusting it over the second. *(Above, left.)*

This picture shows, from the side, the final correct position of the rope behind the ears. *It is not necessary, as so many people think, to pass the ends of the rope into and through the calf's mouth. In fact, if you do this, you will often irreparably damage the calf's jaw and will certainly jeopardise the calf's chances of survival.*

Attach the double rope to a bar, as previously instructed *(above, right)*, and other ropes and bars to both the calf's fore-feet.

Each time the heifer relaxes after straining, exert moderate pressure on the rope around the calf's head. You will find that, in 99 cases out of 100, the head will shoot forward into its correct position. This is one of the few times when you do not pull as the animal strains. (Right.)

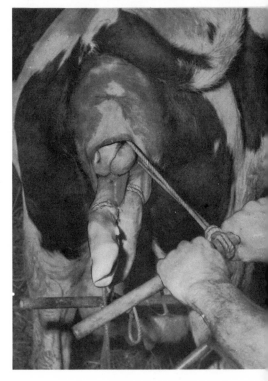

(c) Head out and leg back

A reasonably common malpresentation, especially in heifers, is where the head and one foreleg, or the head alone, is outside the vulva. Frequently, when found, the head and tongue are markedly swollen. *(Top, right—next page.)*

To attempt to pull the calf away in such a situation will, in a heifer, prove difficult or impossible, or at the very least will rip and kill the heifer. If the calf is alive then, most assuredly, it is a job for your veterinary surgeon, because spinal anaesthesia may be absolutely essential before the leg or legs can be brought forward.

However, if the calf is dead, the head excessively swollen, the heifer in acute distress, and a veterinary surgeon not immediately available, then it is possible, on occasion, for an intelligent stockman to manage.

In any case the correct technique, with a dead calf, is as follows:

Having first of all hobbled the heifer to prevent 'splaying', pass the running noose of a nylon calving rope over the top of the calf's head to behind the ears and then tighten the noose. *(Centre, right.)*

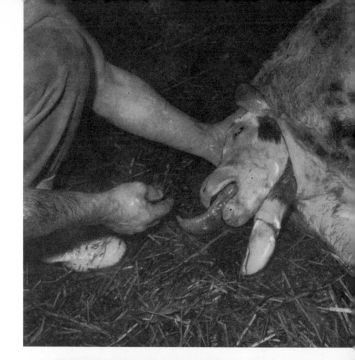

With one man pulling firmly on the rope, cut the calf's head off just behind the ears. For this job, a sharp butcher's knife or bread knife will do, but great care has to be taken not to cut the vulva. It's a good idea to use one hand to hold the membrane and skin of the vulva away from the cutting area during the operation. *(Bottom, right.)*

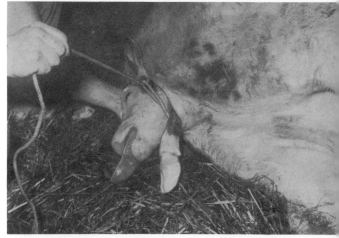

Now push the foetus back into the uterus, pushing particularly between the heifer's strains, and exerting the main pressure with the hand over the stump of the neck. *(Below.)*

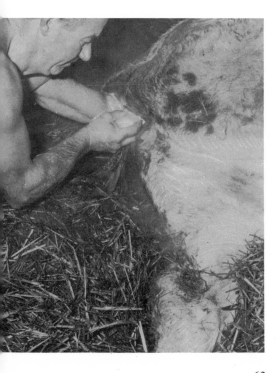

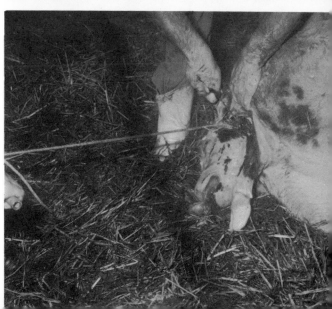

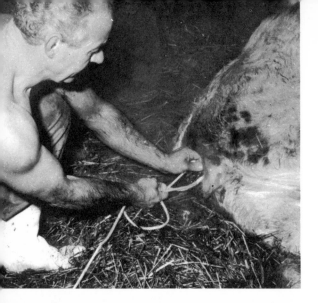

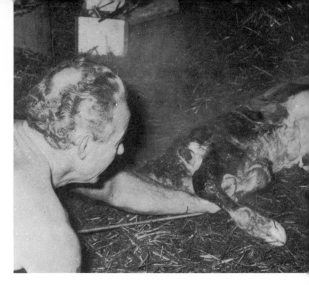

When the foetus is back in the uterus, search for and find the bent back feet or foot. Having done so, introduce the looped end of a calving rope. Pass the noose over the turned back foot, this time to just above the hoof, and tighten it around the calf's pastern. When pressure is exerted on the rope, the foot then bends towards the outside. *(Top left and above.)*

Pull on the rope with one hand and, at the same time, cup the other hand over the bent back claw. This protects the neck of the uterus as the foot comes forward and is an extremely important precaution. *(Centre and bottom, left.)*

When both legs are forward into the passage, rope both feet—this time above the fetlocks. *(Below.)*

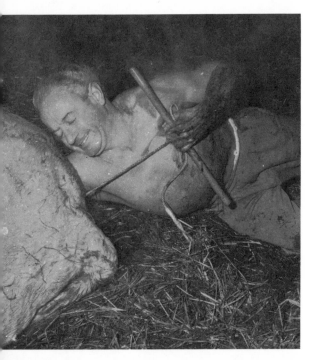

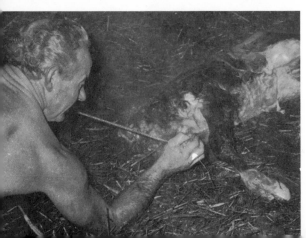

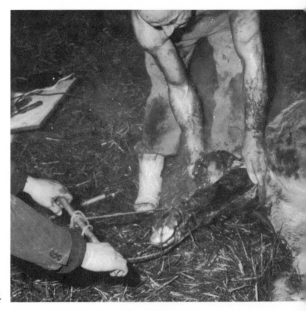

Get an assistant to pull on the legs of the foetus while you use one hand to cover the neck stump to prevent injury to the roof of the vagina. Keep the neck stump covered until it protrudes from the vulva. Once the calf's shoulders are out, the rest is easy.

Exactly the same principles are adopted in all cases where one or both legs are back —the foetus is pushed back as far as possible into the uterus, the foot is roped around the coronet, and one hand is cupped over the foot as it is pulled forward through the cervix. If the foetus is not pushed back, correction is much more difficult and, in a heifer, well nigh impossible.

If the calf is alive, probably only the veterinary surgeon will succeed in delivering it alive. He will most likely use a calculated dose of spinal anaesthetic— usually 4½-5 ccs of a 2% solution. This dose is sufficient to stop the cow straining, but not enough to take away the power of her legs.

The veterinary surgeon will now wash and lubricate the protruding parts of the foetus, get the heifer or cow onto her feet if possible, and gently push the head and leg or the head back into the uterus. He will then bring forward the turned back leg in the manner described.

The spinal anaesthesia may make the cow groggy for an hour or two, but if the floor underneath is sanded or gritted she will come to no harm.

(d) Head down inside uterus

Another simple malpresentation is where the top of the calf's head is presented to the cervix, with the nose and mouth tucked down into the body of the uterus. One or both of the forelegs may also be turned back. *(Below, left and right.)*

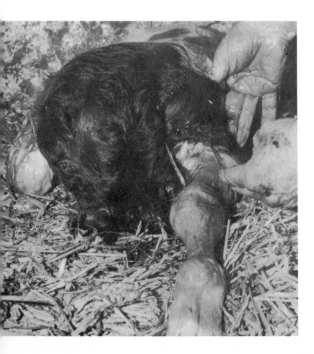

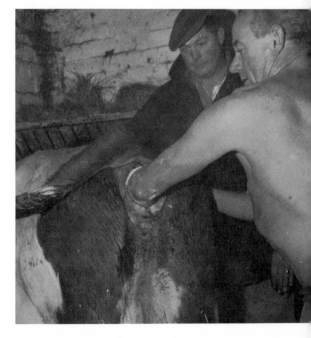

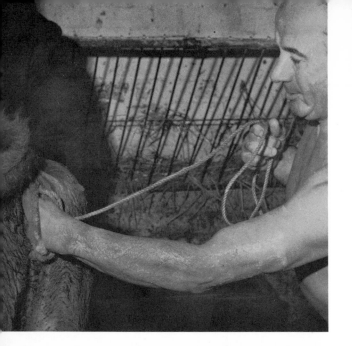

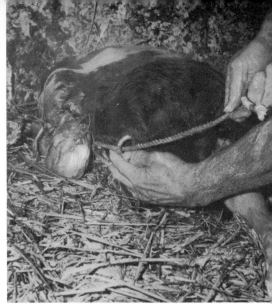

slip the loop up over the fetlock. *(Centre, left.)*

Now introduce the centre part of a looped cord and pass it along the top of the front of the head of the foetus to underneath the lower jaw or chin. *(Below.)*

Place the flat of the left hand on the top of the head of the foetus. As the animal

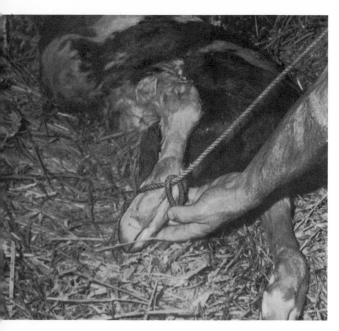

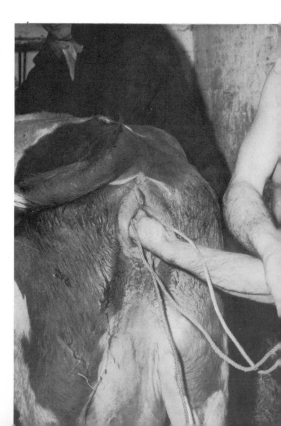

First of all, introduce a running loop of a calving cord and pass it between the side of the head and the inside of the turned back limb. *(Top, left and right.)*

Apply the loop around the calf's coronet and bring the foot forward as instructed in the previous chapter, cupping the hand over the foot as it comes through the cervix. Then, when the foot is forward,

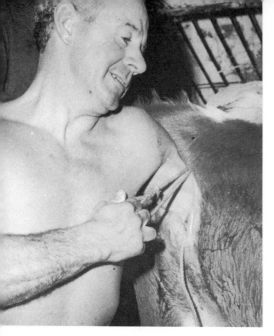 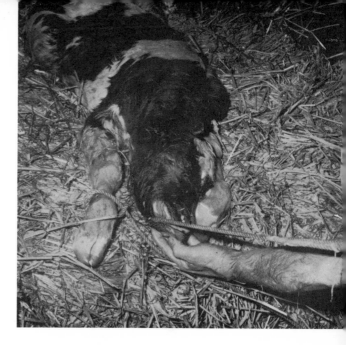

finishes each strain (and never during the strain), push the head back and, at the same time, apply pressure on the ends of the cord. *(Above, left.)*

The calf's head will straighten easily. As it does so, slip the left hand underneath the calf's chin and help the chin over the pelvic brim. *(Above, right.)* If pressure is applied during the straining, there is some danger that the incisor teeth of the foetus may tear or rupture the uterus.

When the position of the head and legs are both corrected, the birth will proceed normally.

(e) Breech presentation

This means simply when the tail end of the foetus is presented at or through the cervix with the hind limbs of the foetus extended downwards, upwards or straight forward into the uterus. *(Below.)*

This presentation is probably one of the most common of all malpresentations. It is one of the easiest to put right if the correct technique is used, and one of the most difficult to attempt if the correct procedure is unknown. The way to deal with a breech presentation is as follows:

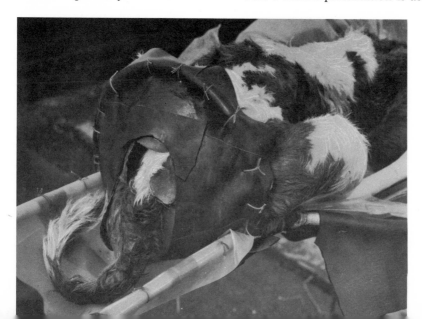

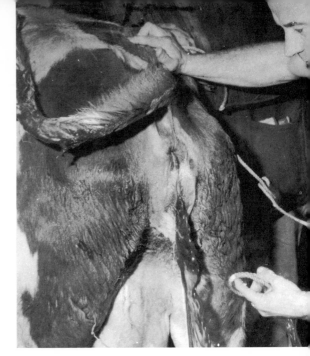

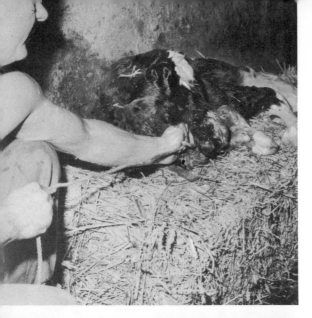

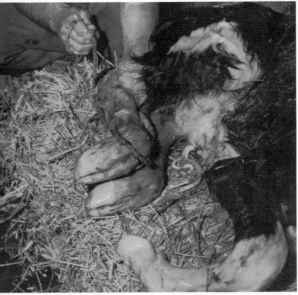

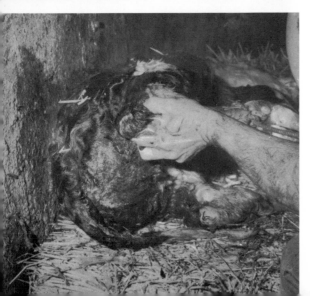

First of all, make a running noose at one end of a calving cord. *(Above.)*

Pass the noose between the turned back hind legs of the calf as far as the nearest foot that can be felt. It may be necessary to hook the hand into the hock joint and pull it forward before a foot can be reached. *(Top, left.)*

Slip the noose over the foot and up to just below the fetlock joint. *(Centre, left.)* In many cases, in heifers particularly, it is better to secure the loop around the pastern–i.e. immediately above the hoof (see diagram illustrating the straightening of the second leg).

Place the flat of the hand underneath the hock of the foetus and push the hock upwards and forwards into the uterus, at the same time maintaining a steady pressure on the roped foot. If a steady pressure is not maintained, the noose of the rope may slip up above the fetlock (as illustrated). When this happens, the foot does not turn backwards correctly and may tear the uterus. *(Bottom, left.)*

The simultaneous pushing forward of the hock and maintenance of steady pressure on the foot, with slight added pressure between the mother's strains, will result in the hind foot shooting forward into the anterior vagina.

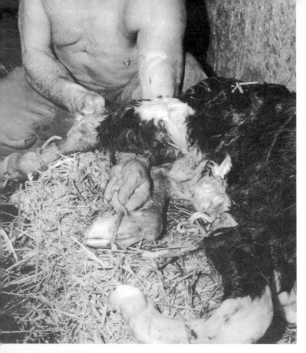

make certain, first of all, that the noose is in the correct position and, secondly, that the front of the foot is not cutting into the wall of the uterus, as it sometimes does just below the cervix.

During the pushing back of the hock steady pressure should be exerted on the rope, but *never excess* pressure. If excess pressure is applied, then obviously there is constant danger of the front of the foot tearing the uterus.

After both legs are straight and forward outside the vulva, move the loops up over the fetlocks before starting to assist. *(Below.)*

Later, when approaching the crisis

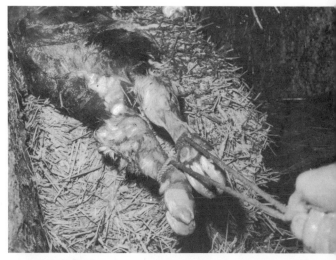

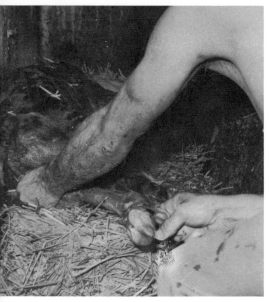

Correction of the second leg is much easier and here you see the correct looping of the cord around the coronet, i.e. just above the hoof. *(Top.)*

Pushing the hock upwards and forward, and simultaneous pulling on the foot, soon results in the straightening of the leg. *(Above and bottom, right.)*

It is a good idea during the straightening, particularly in a heifer, to pass the hand from the hock to the foot occasionally to

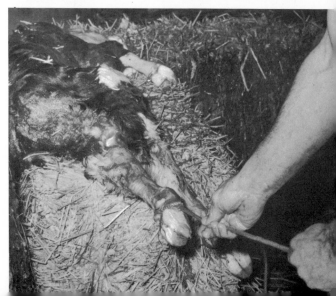

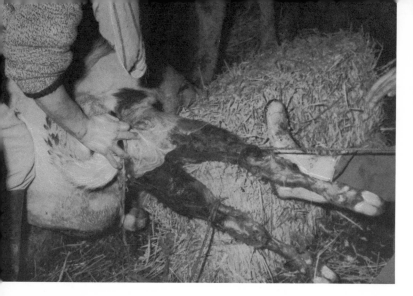 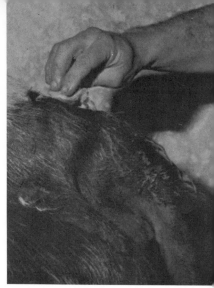

stage (i.e. when the tail part appears outside the vulva), the loops can be fixed *above the hocks* to give the assistant better leverage. Remember, once the hind legs of the 'breach' are straightened, you are dealing with a simple posterior presentation and you should proceed exactly as instructed in the posterior presentation section. *(Above, left.)*

Just occasionally, and particularly with the younger and less experienced veterinary surgeon, spinal anaesthesia may be required before the hocks can be brought forward sufficiently to allow the flat of the hand to get underneath for the upward and forward propulsion. The disadvantage of spinal anaesthesia *(above, right)*, however, is that it interferes with the natural dilation of the cervix.

Less frequently, the joints of the hind legs may be stiffened or 'ankylosed', and it may not be possible to either bend the fetlock or move the hock joint.

In such cases the embryotomy wire has to be introduced around the top of one or both hind legs and the entire stiffened limb or limbs removed. *(Below.)* Usually the removal of only one allows the delivery of the foetus with the remaining ankylosed hind leg still projecting forward.

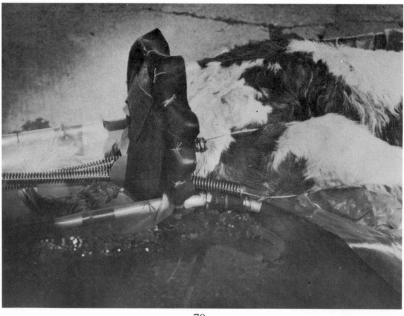

8
The Afterbirth

THE passing of the afterbirth in the cow is the third stage in the natural normal birth. When the afterbirth is retained, therefore, there is always a reason. *(Below, right.)* The causes of the afterbirth retention are:

1. Contagious abortion
2. Vibrio foetus infection
3. Calcium deficiency
4. Magnesium deficiency
5. Blood poisoning, or septicaemia
6. Interference during calving
7. Fatigue after calving

In contagious abortion, which is caused by the germ Brucella abortus, an inflama-

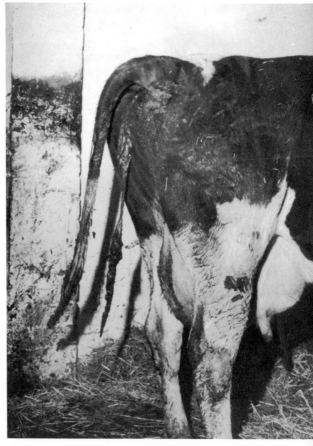

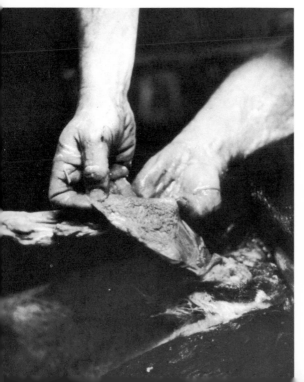

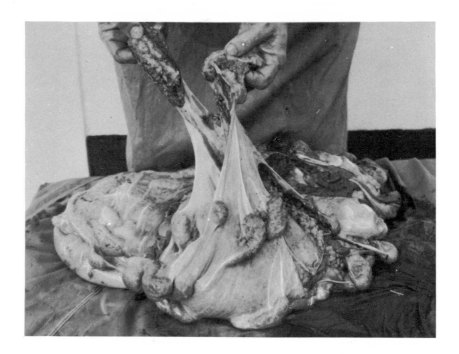

(Above.)

tion of the lining of the uterus or womb causes the afterbirth to adhere to the cotyledons or, as some people call them, 'the roses'. When the inflammation heals, it leaves fibrous or 'scar' tissue between the cotyledons and the cleansing. *(Bottom, left, previous page.)*

Contagious abortion afterbirths can hang for anything up to ten days, or even a fortnight. When they drop, or are removed, the parts that have been attached to the cotyledons have a characteristic yellow colour.

The important thing to remember about retained afterbirths due to the Brucella abortus germ is that the cow does not always calve before her time. This fact is often overlooked.

Remember, therefore, contagious abortion does not always cause abortion—the only sign may be the holding of the afterbirth. Hence, if several cows in the herd are hanging on to their cleansings, blood samples should be taken immediately.

In vibrio foetus infection, the most serious of the bovine venereal diseases, the worst type of retentions occur when the calf is carried to full term. They are often impossible to remove in under ten days, the cotyledons seem to die inside the womb, and invariably you are left with a really sick cow, which stands little chance of breeding again if the veterinary surgeon is not consulted.

When the vibrio cases abort, the afterbirths are also retained and the cotyledons still die. The dead cotyledons subsequently come away with the afterbirth and an evil smell may persist for several weeks. The salvation of such cases lies in the daily injection, for at least a week, of massive doses of antibiotics.

The majority of vibrio cases, of course, don't hold to the bull or break at ten to twelve weeks. Nonetheless, a great many—certainly more than is generally realised—carry their calves to full term and hold their cleansings.

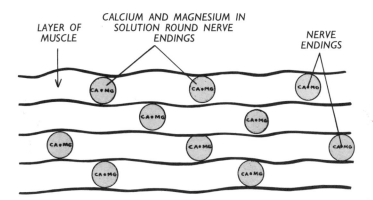

LAYER OF MUSCLE

CALCIUM AND MAGNESIUM IN SOLUTION ROUND NERVE ENDINGS

NERVE ENDINGS

Calcium deficiency and magnesium deficiency cause retention by interfering with the action of the uterine muscle. The explanation of this is that the nerve endings in the muscle are surrounded by a solution containing both these minerals and even a mild shortage of either prevents the uterus from functioning normally. *(Above.)*

In blood poisoning, for example in summer mastitis or in gangrenous mastitis, the germs in the blood excrete waste products called toxins. These toxins damage the muscle fibre and prevent the normal uterine contraction.

When the toxins build up in the system we call the condition 'toxaemia', and this 'toxaemia' is very likely to kill the calf. I'm sure many readers will have seen an acute summer mastitis or an acute 'black garget' leading to a dead calf and a retained afterbirth. *(Right.)*

Interference during calving disturbs the normal uterine contractions and this may lead to retention. Also the damage caused by interference often makes the vulva, vagina, and cervix of the mother so tender and sore that she will make no attempt to void the afterbirth.

Fatigue after calving is occasionally seen after a protracted labour but it is most often manifest when there are twins. Certainly the combined weight of two calves, often well over a 1 cwt, is more than enough

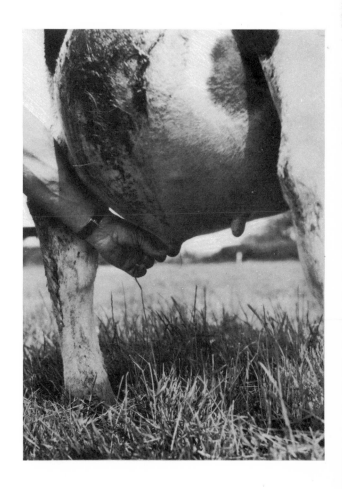

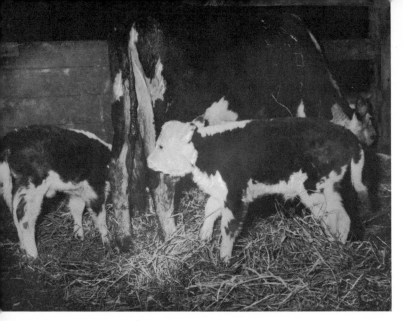

to fatigue any muscle. This is the simple reason why a retained afterbirth is one of the hazards of twin calving. *(Above.)*

What Should be Done?

The most important thing is to safeguard the animal's future breeding potential.

In order to do this, interference should be restricted to an absolute minimum. There is little doubt that a hand moving about inside a uterus for any longer than, say, quarter of an hour at the outside is practically certain to set up a traumatic inflammation and, once this happens, infertility is the likely result.

The cow will certainly lose condition, but my advice is this:

Where there is only an occasional case, clip off the hanging portion of the afterbirth and wash down the hindquarters and udder with hot water, soap and antiseptic. (Below.)

Disregard the portion left inside unless or until the cow goes off her milk or off her food. Then, of course, it is a job for your veterinary surgeon. He will remove the afterbirth or, if the cleansing is not quite ready, he will inject the cow intramuscularly with 5–10 mgm of Stilboestrol and may or may not prescribe a course of antibiotics, depending on how bad the case is.

Where cases of retention are occuring frequently in the herd, the veterinary surgeon should be consulted immediately. He should be able very quickly to pinpoint the predisposing cause and prescribe a cure.

The thing to remember is that an occasional retained afterbirth is inevitable, whereas frequent cases are abnormal and indicate a herd problem.

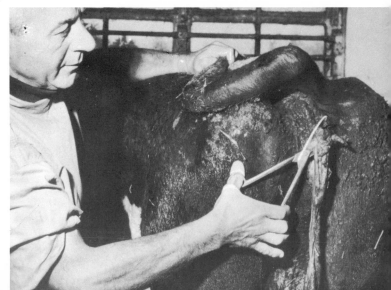

74

9
Spinal Anaesthesia
(Epidural Anaesthesia)

THE USE of spinal anaesthesia is a job for the veterinary surgeon. But none-theless a thorough knowledge of why and how it is used will not only be of value to the veterinary student, but will help the lay reader to more fully understand this aspect of a veterinary surgeon's work.

In spinal anaesthesia local anaesthetic is injected into a space, called the epidural space, which lies at the base of the spinal column at the top of the cow's tail. *(Below.)*

Indications
Spinal anaesthesia is used in:
    (a) Ceasarian section operation
    (b) Prolonged interference
    (c) Prolapsed uterus
    (d) Any local surgery at the back end of
        the cow

In the caesarian section, which is done with the cow standing up, spinal anaes-thesia prevents the cow continually strain-ing and relaxes the uterus when the surgeon comes to handle it.

In difficult cases, where prolonged manipulation or extensive embryotomy (cutting the calf up inside the cow) is required, the spinal anaesthesia not only makes the job infinitely easier for the operator, but goes a long way towards minimising the risk of shock in the patient.

In a prolapsed uterus (see Chapter 12), the spinal anaesthesia is vital because it stops the cow straining and makes the prolapse return very much easier. In local rear-end surgery it removes all pain.

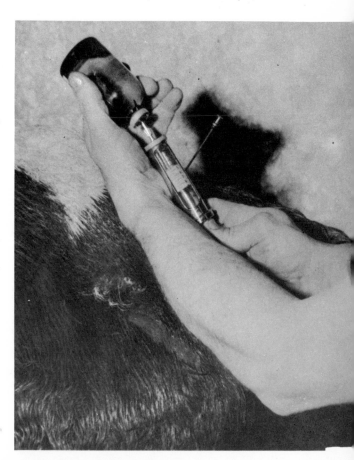

75

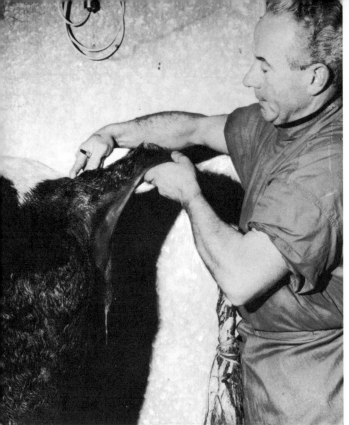

Technique

1. The site generally recommended is the space between the first and second vertebrae of the tail. The site I like best is the space between the fixed end of the spine (the sacrum) and the movable tail. The best way to find the site is to move the entire tail up and down with one hand at the same time feeling with the thumb of the other hand for the space at the first point of movement. *(Left.)*

2. Having established the site, clip all the hair over the area. *(Below, left.)*

3. Now disinfect the site thoroughly with a powerful skin antiseptic. *(Below.)* *right.)* This is tremendously important, since any infection taken into the epidural space (i.e. the space at the end of the spinal cord into which the injection has to be made) can cost the life of the cow.

4. Now take an epidural needle, i.e. a needle specially made for the purpose, which has a central cannulla to avoid

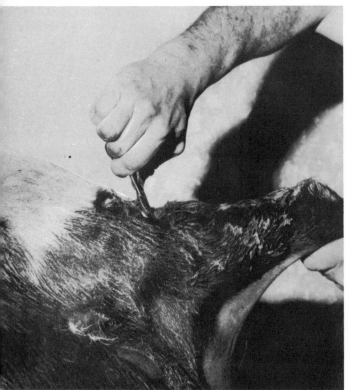

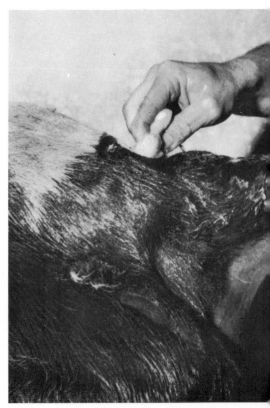

needle blockage. Again, this needle must be absolutely sterile. *(Right.)*

5. Keeping the thumb on the vertebra immediately above the space selected, insert the needle—at an angle of approximately 45°—boldly downwards. The point will come to rest on the floor of the spinal canal. *(Below, right.)*

6. You will know if and when you are in the correct spot when you remove the cannulla from the epidural needle—because then you should hear the hiss of air being sucked into the space in the spinal column. *(Below, left.)*

7. You will further confirm the correctness of your site by the ease with which

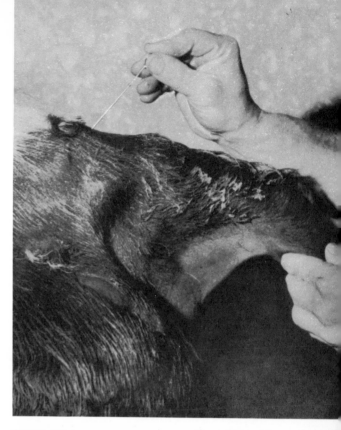

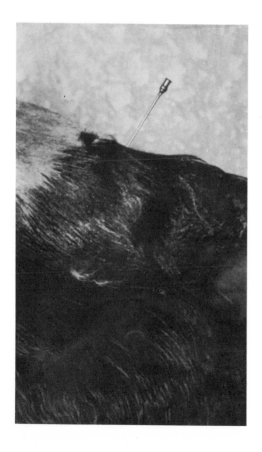

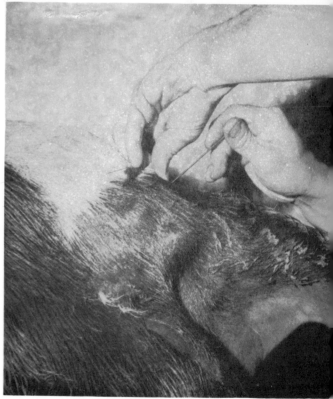

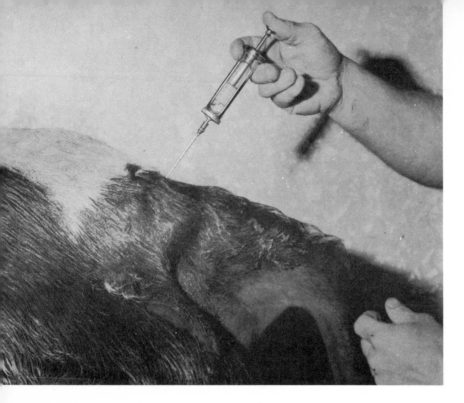

the anaesthetic can be injected. If there is any resistance to the plunger at all, then the needle should be withdrawn and another site tried. *(Above.)*

8. The average dose of local anaesthetic required to stop a cow or heifer straining is around $4\frac{1}{2}$ ccs of a 2% solution of a sterile local anaesthetic. The anaesthetic acts almost immediately and within seconds you should be able to detect a loss of power in the cow's tail. If a larger dose than $4-4\frac{1}{2}$ ccs is given, there is great danger of the cow losing the power of her hind legs. This is undesirable, especially in a caesarian section operation, where the whole job is much easier if and when the patient remains standing.

10
'Torsion' or 'Twist' of the Uterus

OCCASIONALLY, during pregnancy, the uterus containing the calf becomes twisted on its own axis. This causes a 'torsion' or 'twist' of the uterine body just inside the cervix—a torsion which is also manifest in the anterior vagina.

The exact cause of uterine torsion is obscure, but it may be due to a fall or to the excessively vigorous movements of a big calf.

The 'twist' may only be partial or it may be complete, depending on the degree of displacement of the calf. The diagram shows a complete torsion. (*Below.*)

NORMAL

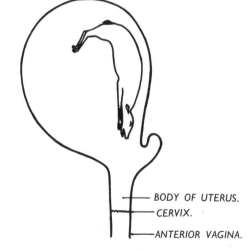

BODY OF UTERUS.
CERVIX.
ANTERIOR VAGINA.

TWISTED

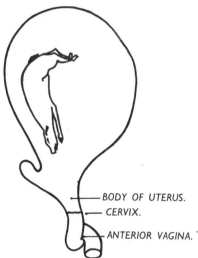

BODY OF UTERUS.
CERVIX.
ANTERIOR VAGINA.

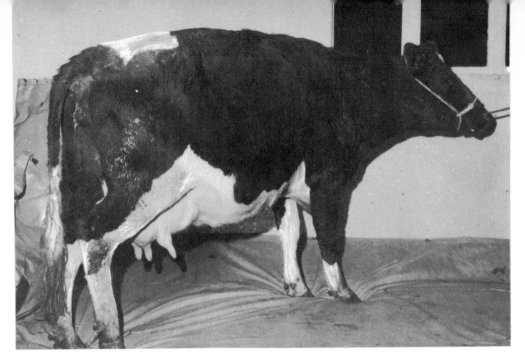

The symptoms are not easy to detect. The cow goes to full term, or perhaps a few days over. She fills her udder and relaxes in the pelvic bones. She then starts showing signs of preliminary labour—mild bouts of labour pain, tail cocking and slight straining.

These symptoms persist and continue without any further progress being made. After twenty-four to forty-eight hours, the cow becomes dejected and off her feed. Her extremities become ice cold. *(Above.)*

What to Do

The diagnosis and treatment of uterine torsion should always be left to the veterinary surgeon, but it's very important that the farmer should spot the condition as early as possible. Obviously the quicker the veterinary surgeon is called the easier his job will be, and the greater his chance of delivering a live calf.

Consequently, in all cases of abnormally protracted first-stage labour, especially in a cow, a vaginal examination should be made. When the hand reaches the anterior vagina a queer tight-banded obstruction will be felt. Further introduction of the hand over the band will reveal the corkscrew torsion. In most cases, as in the one illustrated, the 'twist' will be clockwise in direction. *(Left.)*

If the anterior vagina feels in any way abnormal, you should send for your veterinary surgeon at once.

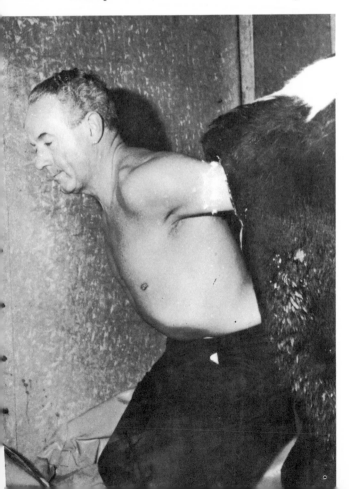

80

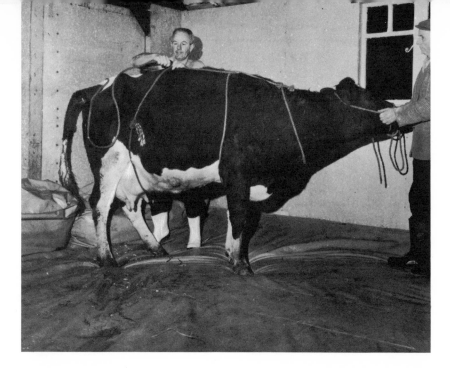

How To Deal With It

The supervision of the correction of a twisted womb must be by the veterinary surgeon. However, since farmers and stockmen will be required to help, a knowledge of what the vet is trying to do should increase the farmer's interest and enthusiasm.

First of all, the cow is roped for casting by 'Reuff's' method—with a fixed noose around the base of the neck and in front of the shoulder (in horned cattle this can be a running noose around the base of the horns); a half-hitch around the cow just behind the elbows; and a second half-hitch around the body of the cow just in front of the udder. *(Above.)*

The cow is cast by pulling tightly on the free end of the rope from directly behind the rear end. The tightening rope acts by exerting pressure on the blood vessels which supply the legs. *(Below.)*

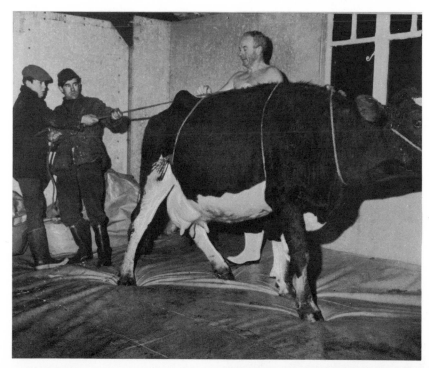

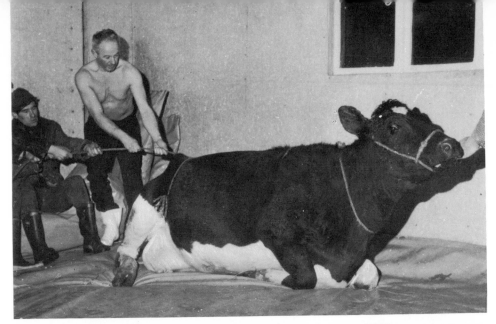

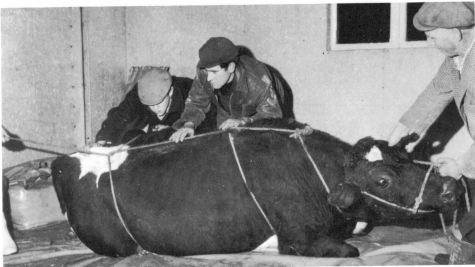

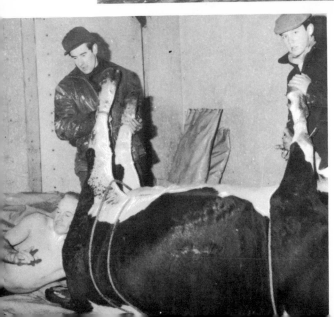

Three-man pressure may be needed, but eventually and certainly the cow will sink down. During the pulling it is essential to have the cow's head held firmly by a halter. In other words, for this job plenty of help is needed—the more the better. *(Top.)*

The cow is now rolled in the direction of the twist—in this case, in a clockwise direction. *(Above.)*

The cow's fore and hind feet are tied, the veterinary surgeon scrubs up and inserts his hand into and through the twist, and the rolling is continued until the cow is on her back. *(Left.)*

82

By keeping his hand in the anterior vagina, the veterinary surgeon can judge if and when the torsion is being untwisted. He can also tell exactly which way to roll and when to stop rolling. *(Right.)*

Considerable mauling and continual turning over may be required before the twist sorts itself out. In some cases, rolling first one way then the other may have to be tried and, occasionally, the cow may have to be rolled over several times in the one direction. Eventually, however, in ninety-nine cases out of a hundred, the torsion will straighten. *(Below.)*

The cow can then be freed, returned to a loose-box, and either calved or left to get on with the job by herself, depending on the degree of dilation of the cervix. Most cases have to be left at least for a time after correction.

If the twist is irreducible, then a caesarian section operation is necessary (see next chapter).

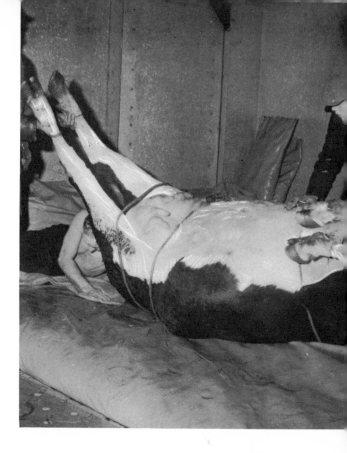

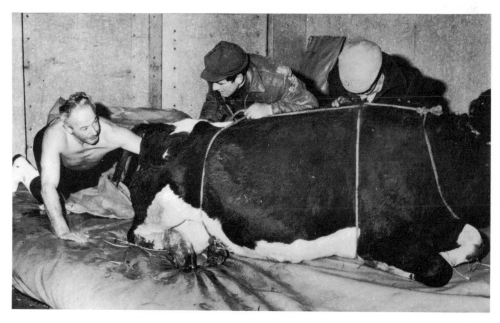

11
Caesarean Section

THE surgical operation of caesarean section in a cow is very much a matter for the veterinary profession. However, I think it is well worth recording a description here, not only for the benefit of both veterinary and agricultural students, but in order that farming readers will understand and appreciate the technique and will, in the comparatively rare cases when the need arises, be able to co-operate more fully with their veterinary surgeon.

The important thing to remember is that, provided the general principles so far outlined in this book are rigidly adhered to, the need for caesarean section will arise only very occasionally.

The indications for operation are:

1. An irreducible 'torsion' of the uterus.

2. A grossly oversized foetus. This is extremely rare but, when it occurs, caesarean is the only answer. The foetus illustrated, for example, weighed 12½ stones and was removed by caesarean section from a six-year-old cow.

3. Certain cases of 'Schiztosoma Reflexus' in a heifer (i.e. an abnormal monstrosity where the foetus is turned inside out). The cases requiring caesarean are where all four feet of the monstrosity are presented.

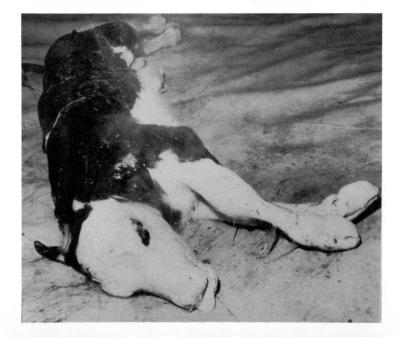

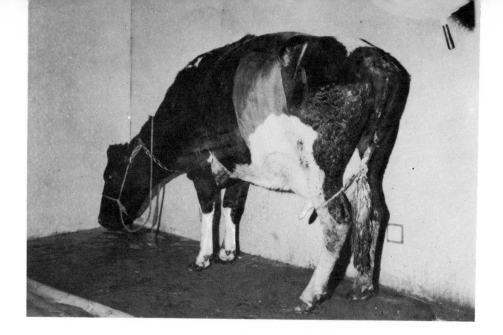

The operation is performed with the patient in the standing position, tied by the neck.

The whole of the left flank area is clipped, shaved and disinfected, and 4 ccs of local anaesthetic is injected into the epidural space as illustrated in the chapter on spinal anaesthesia. This stops the straining and relaxes the uterus.

The cow's tail is tied to the near hind leg and the entire floor area is sanded heavily to prevent the patient slipping about or falling down. *(Above.)*

The site of the operation incision is on the left flank, approximately four inches from and parallel to the last rib, and extending over a distance of between 13 to 15 inches. *(Right.)*

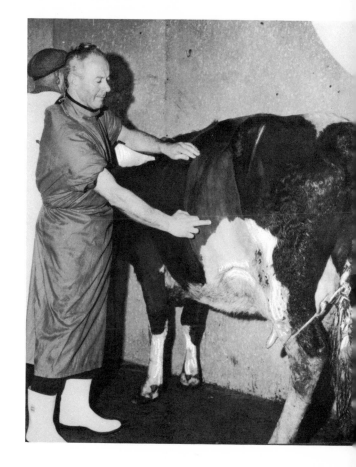

The Anaesthetic

Since the operation is done with the cow standing, local anaesthesia has to be used —there are two alternative methods.

First of all a nerve block which produces regional anaesthesia of the entire flank. This technique is called 'Paravertebral Anaesthesia' and comprises the blocking of the main nerve branches as they come off the spinal column. A long needle, and considerable practice and skill, are re-

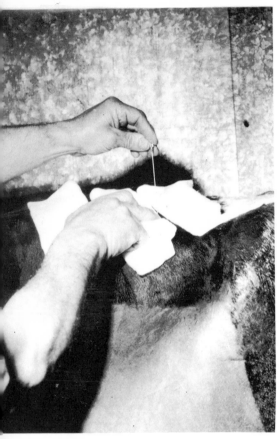

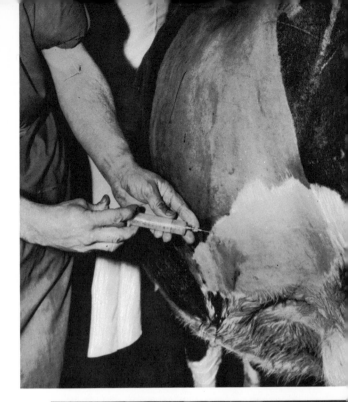

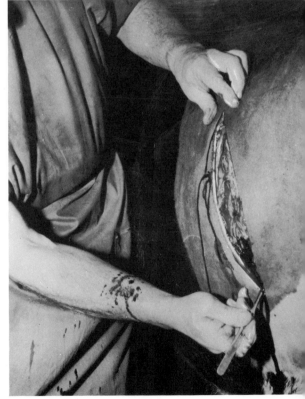

quired to perfect this technique. *(Above.)*

The other, and more widely used, method is the local infiltration of the anaesthetic over and through the entire site of incision. For this job more anaesthetic is required, but many veterinary surgeons prefer the infiltration method, probably because the paravertebral block has occasionally let them down, resulting in an upset patient and considerable loss of time. *(Top, right.)*

The Operation
The anaesthetic takes approximately five minutes to produce its effect. The 13–15 inch incision is then made through the skin, parallel to and approximately four inches from the last rib. *(Below, right.)*

The incision is continued through the two and three layers of muscle—two layers at the top and three layers at the bottom of the wound. *(Right.)*

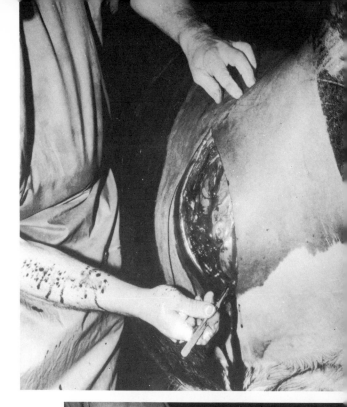

The peritoneum, or white glistening membrane which lines the abdominal cavity and encloses its contents, is now exposed. *(Below, left.)*

The peritoneum is cut with a pair of scissors, the left hand holding the abdominal contents in position while the right-hand and arm are coated with antibiotic. This is not only an aseptic precaution, but the oily base of the antibiotic serves as a lubricant and makes manipulation much easier inside the abdominal cavity. *(Below, right.)*

Both hands and arms have been coated in antibiotic, the uterus has been brought forward and upwards to the mouth of the

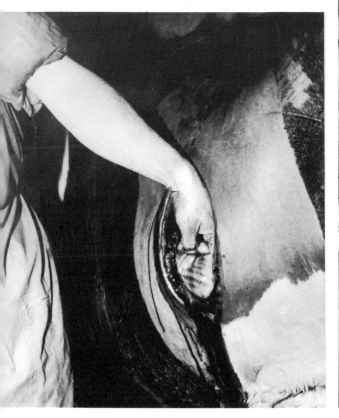

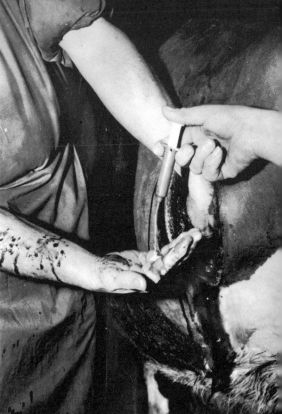

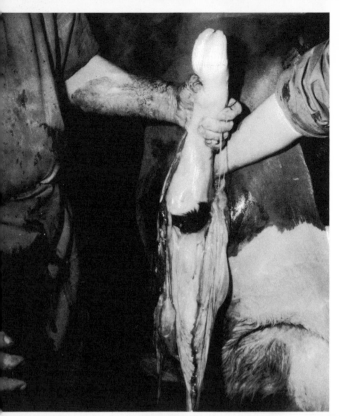

wound, an incision has been made through the uterine wall, and one hind foot of the calf has been brought out. This is held firmly to keep the uterus in position while the incision in the uterine wall is enlarged. *(Left.)*

Both hind feet are now out and are held rigidly while the uterine incision is enlarged still further to allow the free passage of the calf. *(Bottom, left.)*

The calf is now lifted out as quickly as possible. Any delay at this stage will result in death of the calf from suffocation, because the navel cord will break sooner than in normal vaginal delivery. *(Bottom, right.)*

The afterbirth is removed and the wound in the uterus is closed by a single catgut continuous 'lembert' suture, i.e. a stitch which brings the opposing surfaces of the

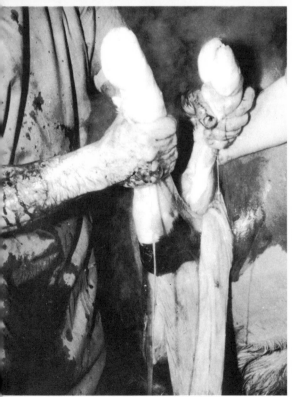

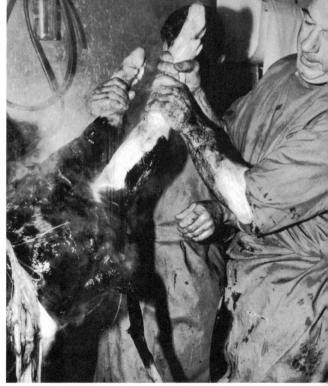

wound into close apposition. *(Right.)*

The surgeon has to work very quickly because the uterus contracts rapidly. If, as occasionally happens, the afterbirth cannot be removed, there is no need to worry because it will be voided subsequently per vagina in the usual way.

The peritoneum and muscles are now closed by a series of straightforward continuous catgut sutures. *(Below, left.)*

Finally, the skin wound is closed by a series of silk mattress sutures. These external stitches will be removed in ten days, but the internal catgut will be absorbed after approximately 20 days. *(Below, right.)*

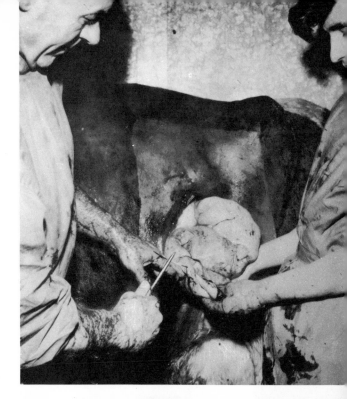

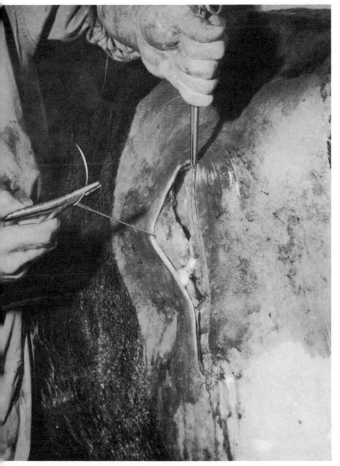

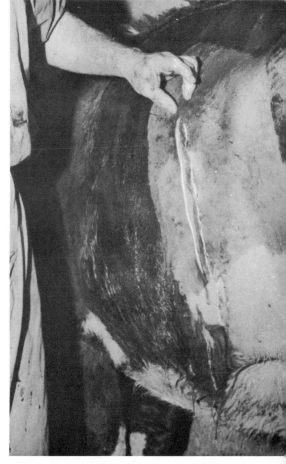

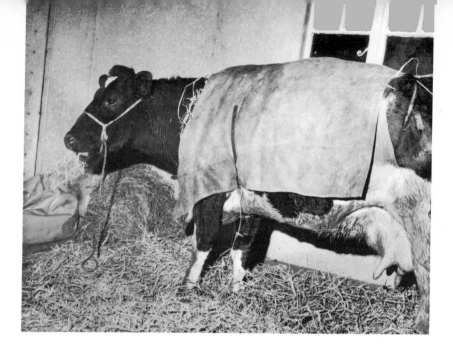

A sight which delights every surgeon—the patient ten minutes after the operation—rugged up and contentedly munching hay. *(Above.)* In other words this operation, spectacular and gory though it may appear, is successful in the majority of cases and should be embarked upon, when absolutely necessary, with the greatest of confidence.

One last word of advice on bovine obstetrics. Perhaps the best way of all to minimise calving difficulties in any breed is to refrain from using, on heifers, a Friesian or a Charolais bull.

12
The Problem of Prolapse

(a) Prolapsed cervix and vagina

THE PROLAPSED CERVIX usually occurs when the cow is heavy in calf. In the early stages, the cow shows only a portion of the cervix and this mainly when lying down. Later, the prolapse may become an angry-looking red mass, even though when the cow stands up the prolapse still disappears.

When the calf gets close to full term—or if, as often happens, the urinary bladder becomes incorporated inside the prolapse—then the prolapse stays out and gets bigger and angrier looking the longer it is left without attention. What happens is that the ligaments and muscles which normally hold the vagina and bladder in position become stretched or torn due to the weight of the extended uterus. *(Below.)*

What To Do
The main thing is not to panic—a cow which 'shows her reed' before calving very rarely prolapses the cervix, vagina or uterus after calving. *Despite this fact, it is unwise to keep the cow for subsequent breeding, since the trouble will reappear earlier in the following pregnancy and will be correspondingly more difficult to deal with.*

How To Deal With It
This is definitely a job for the veterinary surgeon. He will probably use spinal anaesthesia, then he will wash and dry the prolapse, dress with a suitable antibiotic

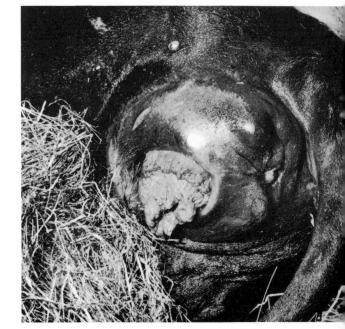

or sulpha dressing, and replace and suture in position.

He will most likely use a deep mattress suture (or stitch)—at least, this is the one I like best. Using strong silk or nylon, he will pass his needle as deeply as possible through both sides at the top of the vulva (taking a good 'bite' of the skin alongside).

Then he will bring the needle to the bottom of the vulva and, taking great care not to include the urethral orifice (i.e. the hole leading into the bladder), he will pass his needle right back through both sides, this time in the opposite direction and again as deeply as possible. *(Right.)* He will then tie a reef knot on the side of the original entry of the needle.

This stitch will last for at least 14 days but, after that time, it may have to be renewed if the patient still hasn't calved.

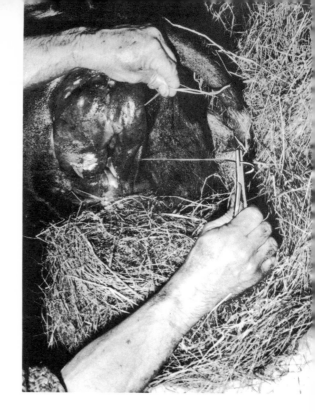

(b) Prolapsed uterus (or womb)

Occurrence and Cause

This condition is not common. In fact, many farmers go through life without a single case and those who do see one often regard it as a 'once-in-a-lifetime' experience. *(Right.)*

However, there are exceptions and a number of cases may occur on the same farm. The explanation of this may lie in the chief predisposing cause in cows— calcium deficiency. A lack of calcium causes the tone of the uterine neck (or cervical) muscles to be lost and this allows the whole uterus to come away.

What appears to happen in many cases is that the milk fever associated with the calcium deficiency makes the cow lie flat on her side, the rumen blows up and, when the blown, constipated, calcium-deficient cow strains to pass dung, the abdominal

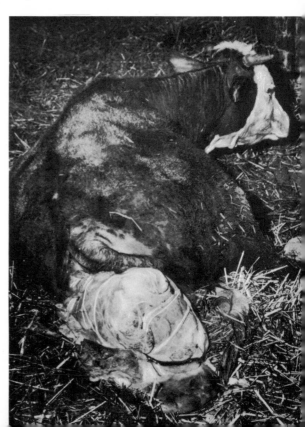

pressure pushes the uterus through the relaxed cervix.

Obviously, the incidence of calcium deficiency will vary from area to area and from herd to herd.

Does this hold good with heifers? The answer must be no. I have yet to see a uterine prolapse in a first-calver where the patient has shown any signs of milk fever.

The cause here appears to be a simple turning inside out of the tip of the pregnant uterine horn. During the final expulsion of the calf, the tip of the horn folds inward on itself, rather like the toe of a sock being turned inside out. Once this happens, the continuing uterine contractions increase the eversion and eventually push the lot out.

Nonetheless, I have found it wise to inject calcium into heifers as well as cows before attempting the prolapse return.

The predisposing cause in first-calvers is often excessive manual pulling at calving time. By exerting a continual high-pressure pull, the uterus is not allowed to relax and fall back into its normal position between contractions. Obviously, this is

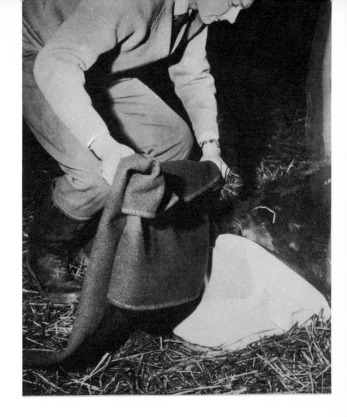

likely to cause the tip of the horn to turn inward on itself.

How To Recognise
Whenever there is a huge red mass, dotted over with large lumps or 'cotyledons', protruding from the vulva after calving, you have a prolapsed uterus. Often the cleansing is still attached to the cotyledons (or 'roses' as they are sometimes called).

The sight of this gives one a lasting knowledge of how the afterbirth is attached to the uterus. *(Bottom, left.)*

First Aid
First-aid measures are simple. *(Above.)*

After phoning an urgent call through to your veterinary surgeon (and these cases get priority from us), all that is necessary is to keep the prolapse as clean and as warm as possible. A clean sheet and blanket are quite adequate, but hot water bottles and hot towels are better.

If the cow is in a yard, move all the other cattle away from her lest they trample on the prolapse. If she is tied up in a shippon,

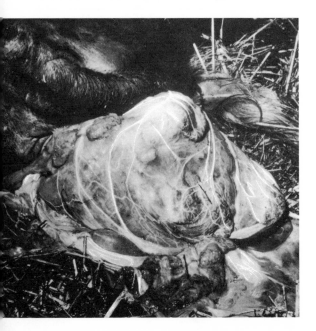

prompt action is even more urgent—get a man to stand protectively over the prolapse while the two neighbouring cows are turned out. I've seen several uteri ruptured by the feet of neighbouring cows. *(Right.)*

Don't whatever you do, attempt to push the prolapse back, because you'll kill the cow (or yourself) for sure.

If you must exercise your genius, and you have a flutter valve and some calcium handy, give one bottle of calcium underneath the skin, high up one handsbreadth

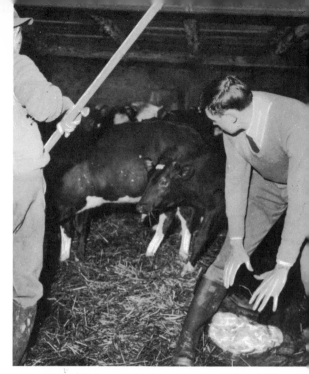

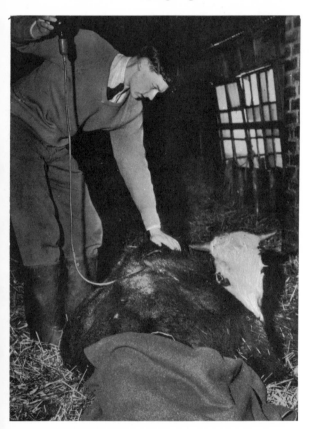

behind the shoulder. *(Above.)* Rub it well away, then sit back and wait for your veterinary surgeon.

Uterine prolapse return is one job where everything is needed—scientific knowledge, professional skill, experience, im-

provisation and a very considerable amount of physical strength. The use of spinal anaesthesia, antibiotics, absolute cleanliness, special drugs to contract and protect the uterus, non-irritant lubricants, and a technique devised by trial and error throughout the years, enables the veterinary surgeon to save the vast majority of uterine prolapse cases.

The technique which I have found best —and this information is for the veterinary reader, particularly—is as follows:

Check and lay out all tools for job, and check on coverage and warmth of uterus. *(Below.)*

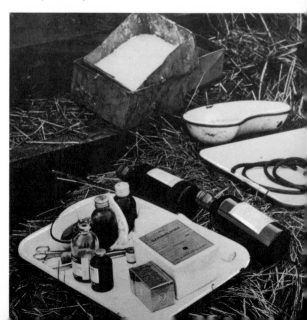

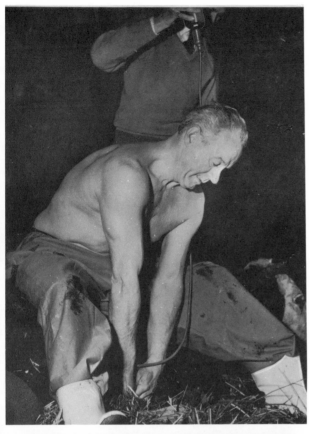

Give calcium injection intravenously, and subcutaneously also if the owner hasn't already done this. *(Left.)*

Inject approximately 5 ccs of a 2% solution of local anaesthetic into the epidural space. This will stop the animal straining against the return of the prolapse. *(Below, right.)*

Inject a dose of muscle relaxant intravenously or intramuscularly. *(Below, left.)* This will relax particularly the muscles around the vulva and vagina. An intramuscular injection of an extract of the pituitary gland may be given to contract and reduce the prolapse size.

After five minutes, roll the animal onto a sleeper or beam. *(Top of next page.)* If this is not practicable and if the cow is in a cowshed, pull her head end round into the grip and roll her hind end over on to the bed.

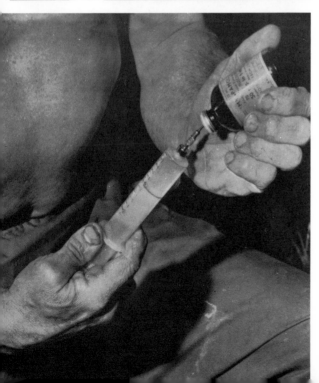

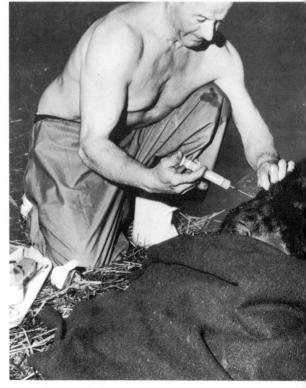

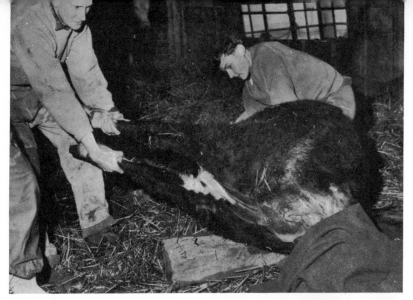

Either of these precautions is essential for two reasons. Firstly it allows the spinal anaesthetic to spread and act more completely and, secondly, almost as important, it throws the weight of the abdominal contents forward, leaving more room for the prolapse return and making the return infinitely easier.

Insert a pastry board or tray under-

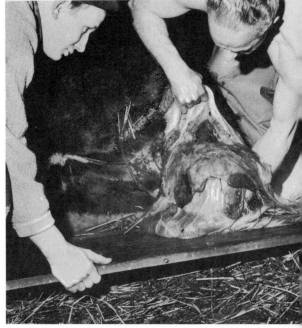

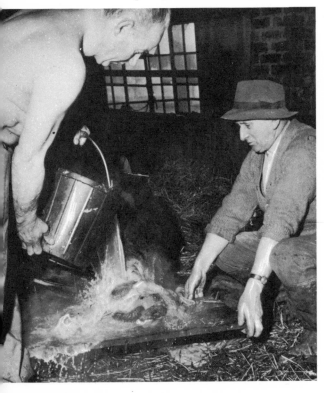

neath the prolapse, with an assistant holding the ends of the board on either side. (*Above.*) This is an excellent hint, because it means that the operator does not have to hold the weight of the baulk while he is pushing it back.

Wash the prolapse thoroughly (*left*), and dress with antibiotic sulpha powder and lubricant. Again, the best lubricant is soap flakes.

Return the prolapse slowly and carefully, using the flat of both hands and working continuously close to the vulva.

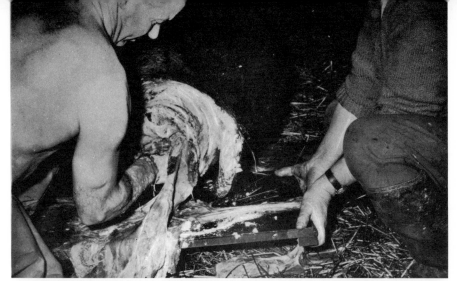

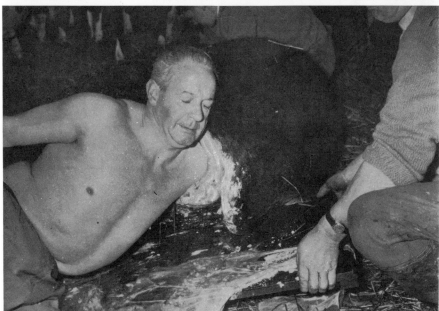

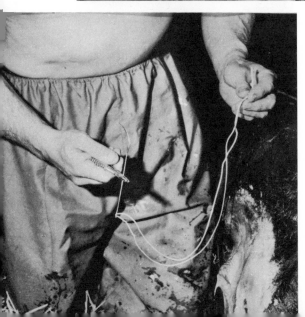

If the cow stands up during the process the job is much easier, provided the assistants continue to take the weight of the board. *(Top.)*

When the prolapse is back in the abdominal cavity, it is vitally important to make sure that the horns of the uterus are invaginated completely. If this is not done, the patient will strain the prolapse out again. Once the prolapse is returned correctly, it never comes out again. *(Above.)*

Despite this, it is always wise to insert a deep mattress suture as illustrated in previous chapter. *(Left.)*

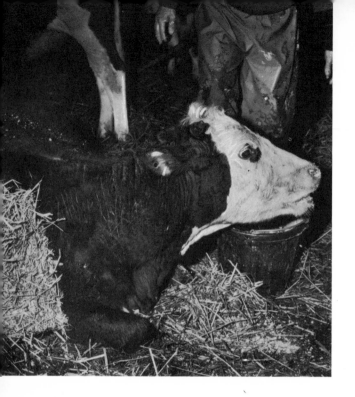

A three-day course of intramuscular antibiotic completes the treatment and ensures the maximum chance of the cow subsequently holding to the bull. To my mind, this is very important. *(Below.)*

Two final important practical points:

Never scrap a cow after a uterine prolapse—rarely if ever will the cow evert her uterus twice. This may well be due to adhesions being set up inside after the mauling of the first return, adhesions which anchor the uterus in its correct place.

Never—and I repeat never—resort to excess pulling when calving a heifer. Remember, one man and patience are all that are needed, assisting only when necessary, and then only when the animal strains.

The two main enemies of the veterinary surgeon are shock and bowel prolapse. The shock syndrome is most often seen in older cows, or where the uterus has been out for a long time.

Usually such patients offer little or no resistance to the prolapse return, but only rarely do they survive. They refuse to eat or drink after the operation, their extremities are ice cold, and often they breathe heavily or grunt ominously. I think such cases are better butchered, though occasionally I have pulled the odd one 'back from the grave' with a blood transfusion.

When the bowel comes out inside the uterus, then the replacement really is a dreadful, heartbreaking, and often impossible job, though few veterinary surgeons will give up without a long and exhausting try.

Occasionally gangrene has set in, but even then something can be done. The gangrenous uterus can be amputated with reasonable hope of success.

I always find that if a cow or heifer will eat and/or drink after a prolapse return or amputation, she will live and do well. If she won't show any interest, she rarely survives. *(Above.)*

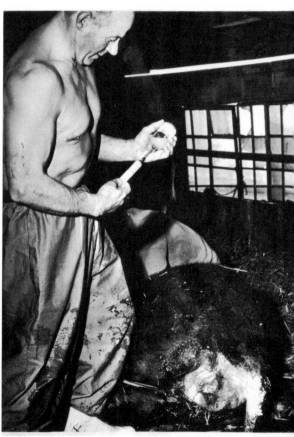

13
Hydrops Amnii

(Uterine Dropsy)

THIS IS a condition where the foetal membranes surrounding the calf accumulate a massive quantity of oedematous or dropsical fluid. *(Below, left.)*

Symptoms
For a considerable time the cow looks as though she is carrying twins.

Towards the end of the gestation period the uterus and abdomen become so grossly distended that the cow has great difficulty in rising or walking about. *(Below, right.)* She may start to grunt, and go off her food. Her extremities become ice-cold.

Treatment
If the condition can be diagnosed early enough, there are two alternatives— immediate slaughter for salvage or the termination of the pregnancy.

The latter can be done by hormone injections or by opening up the cervix and rupturing the membranes.

If the cow does go to full term, there is a very grave danger of severe shock when she loses the massive fluid content of the uterus. Salvage slaughter at this later stage, however, is rarely economical because the oedema has often extended into the carcase.

Early diagnosis and prompt co-operation with your veterinary surgeon are therefore vital.

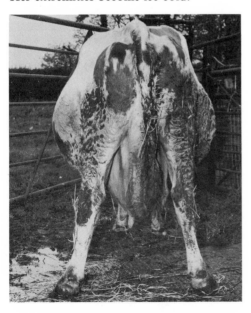

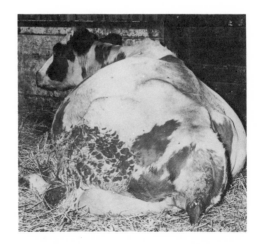

99

14
Infertility

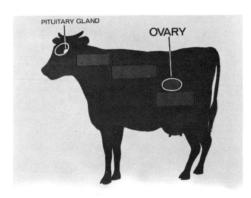

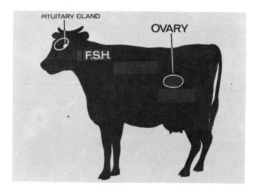

BEFORE ONE can. begin to understand the problem of infertility, a knowledge of the simple physiological function of the cow's reproductive system is absolutely essential.

First of all the pituitary gland, a small gland at the base of the brain, secretes a 'follicle-stimulating' hormone. This stimu-

lates the production of 'follicles' in the ovaries—i.e. small cavities which contain the eggs or ova. *(Above and below, left.)*

Once every three weeks the ovaries themselves manufacture a hormone called oestrin. This produces the oestrus or heat period. *(Below, right.)*

Towards the end of the heat period the

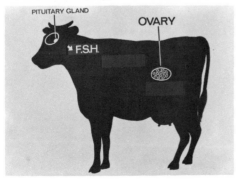

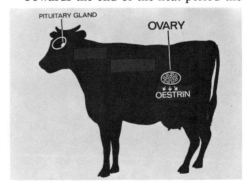

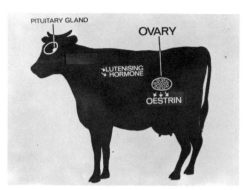

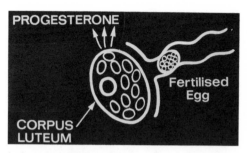

in its passage through the pituitary gland it stops the production of the follicle-stimulating hormone. *(Above.)*

This breaks the natural sexual cycle and

pituitary gland gets going again and this time secretes another hormone, called a luteinising hormone. *(Above.)* This is carried via the bloodstream to the ovaries where it causes the follicle or follicles to rupture, thereby releasing the egg or eggs which drop down into the oviducts or fallopian tubes. There they await fertilisation by the spermatozoa either from the bull or from A.I. *(Below.)*

If conception does take place, a small

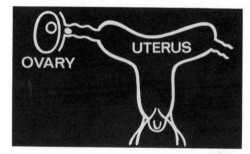

the cow does not come into season again until the ovary sheds the corpus luteum, usually about the eighth or ninth day after calving. *(Above.)*

Conception (or fertilisation of the egg by the sperm) takes place in the upper part of the oviduct. Three or four days later the fertilised egg comes down into the uterus where it starts to grow into the foetus. *(Below.)* In 30 to 40 days after fertilisation, the foetus becomes attached to the cotyledons which grow from the lining of the uterine wall.

Any factor which interferes with any

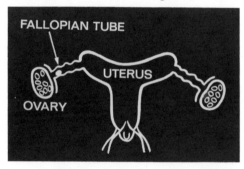

body, called the corpus luteum, develops in the ovary *(below)* and manufactures yet another hormone, called progesterone. The progesterone gets into the blood and,

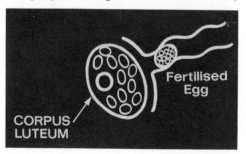

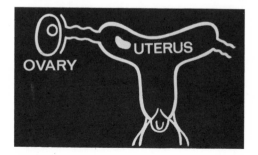

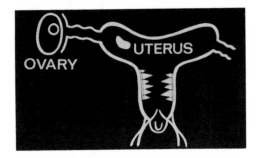

stage of this normal sexual cycle can produce infertility.

Obviously an infection in the uterus or fallopian tubes will 'gum up' the works, an infection could be caused by the contagious abortion bug—the *Brucella abortus*—or by one of the venereal diseases—trichomoniasis, vibrosis or coital exantheima ('bull burn'). Luckily the use of A.I. has largely reduced these venereal diseases to a minimum. *(Above.)*

One of the commonest infections is a fungus which causes 'mycotic abortion'. This fungus gets to the cattle in mouldy hay or mouldy straw, so if we have a wet summer and a bad harvest don't feed the mouldy fodder to your breeding stock. Keep the best hay only for the in-calvers and the milkers, the mouldy hay can be used up on the store cattle. I can assure you mouldy fodder can be more dangerous to your herd than either brucellosis or venereal disease, so be careful. This very simple hint can save a lot of money. *(Right.)*

Undoubtedly, nowadays, nearly all the infertility problems I have to deal with are not due to infection and many of these present a real headache. The scientists describe them broadly as 'non-infectuous *infertility*', but I've often described them in language a great deal more expressive.

One of the most common 'breaks' in the sexual cycle is the condition of anoestrus, where the heifer or cow fails to come into season. This is due merely to a low or negative output of follicle-stimulating hormone.

In the dairy cow the cause is usually a high milk yield on a comparatively low protein diet especially when the cow is still growing, which she does up to her third calf. Occasionally it is due to a relative mineral deficiency—deficiency of phosphorus or of the trace elements copper, cobalt and manganese.

In the heifer it can be caused by malnutrition, mineral deficiency, parasitism, or cold or lack of shelter. In fact, any debilitating factor or disease, such as Johne's disease, can lead to anoestrus.

The same factors—especially the high milk yield on the low protein diet—can interfere with the production of the luteinising hormone. When this happens the heat periods last for up to several days and the cows rarely hold to the bull.

The simple answer to these problems is a professional consultation with your local veterinary surgeon as soon as possible.

But the biggest headache of all—one that is becoming an increasing nightmare to progressive dairy farmers and veterinary surgeons alike—is the condition of 'cystic ovaries'.

The cystic condition develops when ovulation does not take place, i.e. when either the egg doesn't develop correctly within the follicle or more commonly

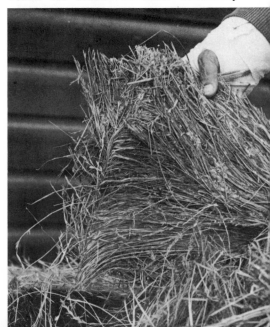

when the follicle fails to rupture when the egg is ripe. Again, this is due to disfunction of the pituitary gland leading to a lack of the luteinising hormone.

What causes cystic ovaries? Without a doubt the most common stress factor producing this ailment is a high milk yield coupled with a comparatively low plane of nutrition. This, I am certain, is the reason why we are seeing more and more cystic ovaries on modern dairy farms.

The trouble is that, in many cases, the cows have been bred for high milk production and are now expected to produce the high yields either on grass or on grass products subsidised only by low protein cereals. Very often cysts first develop in the two or three months after the third lactation when the cow is reaching its peak production.

Just occasionally cysts can be hereditary, and the trouble can also be caused by a deficiency of the trace element, manganese, which gets locked up in the soil when too much nitrogen is used to boost the young spring grasses. The deficiency persists in the silage and hay and builds up as the winter progresses and other stress factors such as cold and exposure take a hand.

But nearly always the cause is the persistent taking of the gallons out of the pint pots, so my advice is to use commercial cattle and be content with lower yields.

CARE OF THE CALF

15
Calf Housing

(a) The floor of the calf pens

THIS ASPECT of calf housing has to date received probably the least attention of all and yet, to my mind, it is of vital importance.

Again and again, I walk into calf pens where the floor conditions are akin to a soggy bog. Again and again, I ask farmers how they'd like to lie and sleep on such a bed. I make it clear that they, too, would get pneumonia and scour if they had to—and yet I have the greatest difficulty in persuading anyone to do anything about it. *(Below, left.)*

This is just crazy, particularly when calf losses now amount to over ten million pounds per year and a single calf can be worth over £40. It is all the more crazy when one considers how easy it is on any farm to provide a clean dry bed by improvisation or by the expenditure of a minimum of capital.

How to Get a Dry Bed

(a) *A layer of ashes*—at least 9-12 inches thick—underneath the bedding. *(Right.)* In addition there should be a drainage fall towards the entrance on the floor underneath, but the drainage fall in itself, without ashes, is completely inadequate.

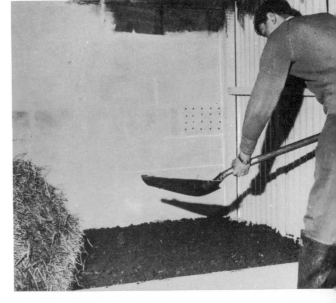

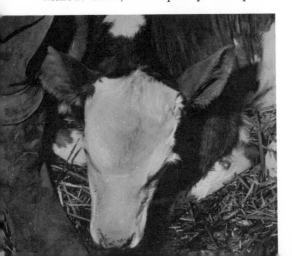

The great advantage of the layer of ashes is that it can be used anywhere and costs virtually nothing.

(b) *Spaces in the floor to allow the urine to drain away*—This is not a slatted floor because the drainage spaces are no more than one quarter of an inch across and the distance between the spaces should be at least eight inches. The floor is laid in concrete strips with a fall of at least two inches from the back of the pen to the front, with a drainage channel underneath which can be flushed through easily.

This type of floor works extremely well and the bedding remains remarkably dry. *(Right.)*

(c) *Slatted floors*—Personally I do not like slatted floors because they lead to misshapen legs but, provided the calves are being kept on them for only a limited period of time—say a six-week maximum —and provided abundant quantities of straw can be used and replaced daily, then slats are infinitely better for calves than the traditional floors, particularly during the susceptible first few weeks of life. The slats can be of wood or concrete and the spaces should not exceed half an inch.

The slats illustrated are on a platform which fits the individual calf pen and which

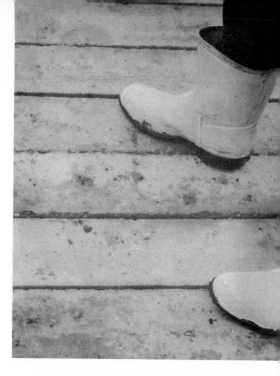

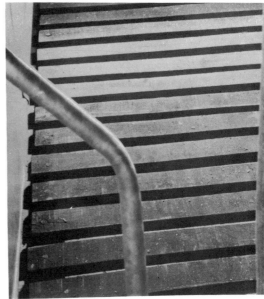

can easily be removed for sterilisation purposes. *(Above.)*

(d) *Sawdust bedding*—For calves where there are no ashes under the bed, no spaces in the floor, and no slats, sawdust provides a reasonable, consistently-dry bedding, provided it is renewed in considerable thickness at least every other day. *(Left.)*

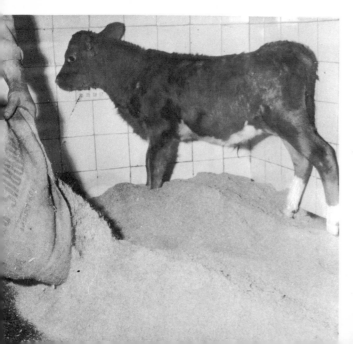

108

Why a Clean Dry Floor

First of all, because it goes a long way towards preventing joint-ill. During the first three days of life, and particularly during the vital first 24 hours, the navel presents a patent entry for infection and, obviously, dirty soaking-wet bedding is much more likely to harbour infection than a clean dry bed. *(Right.)*

Secondly, persistent lying in damp dirty conditions is bound to lower the calves' resistance and predispose to the flare-up of scour, pneumonia and calf diptheria.

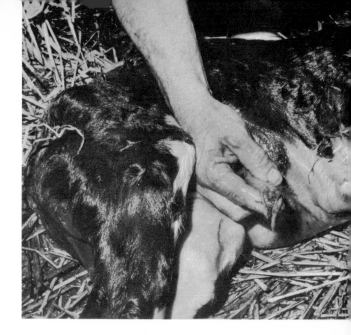

(b) The ideal environment

Environment is all important to calves, particularly to young calves up to the age of three weeks, because during the first three weeks of life the heat-regulating centre in the calf's brain does not function properly. This means that the calf is not able to adapt itself to sudden changes of temperature. Consequently, if it is exposed to such sudden changes, its entire resistance is lowered and it becomes susceptible to all the infectious diseases—scour, pneumonia, joint-ill, calf diptheria, etc.

The important thing, therefore, is to maintain the young calf at a constant temperature, or as near a constant temperature as possible.

This explains why calves born and reared outside rarely contract disease—theirs is a constant environment and any change in temperature is rarely sudden. In other words, it doesn't really matter what temperature the calf is kept at, so long as the temperature remains the same. Obviously, of course, the housed calf will grow and do better if the constant temperature is a reasonably warm one. *(Below.)*

The prevalent causes of rapid temperature changes in the average calf pen are draughts, uninsulated roofs and walls, and

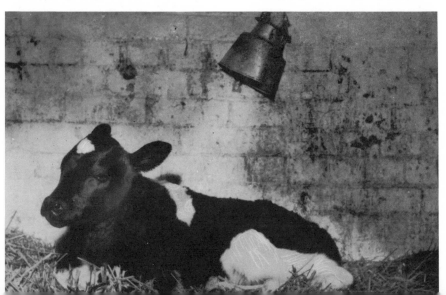

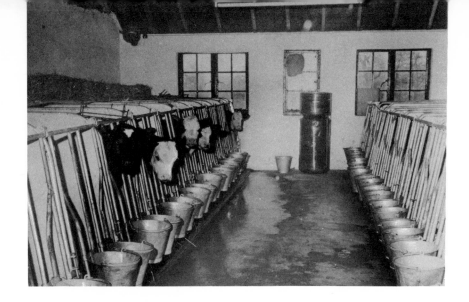

excessively high roofs which provide too much air space per calf. Obviously, therefore, in providing a suitable environment for housed calves, all these faults have to be eliminated.

Tumbledown multipurpose buildings, so often used for calf rearing, are literally 'death traps'.

An Ideal Environment

For this you require thermostatically-controlled air-conditioning within an insulated building, with the maintenance of a temperature of around 60°. This is not by any means as difficult to obtain as it sounds.

In the ideal house illustrated, for example, the insulation is provided by hollow-brick tiles underneath the floor, traditional cavity walls, and a loft overhead. The air conditioning plant, although installed by experts, was extremely reasonable in cost and the entire house was built by casual labour. Ample light is provided by a range of large windows facing south.

Perhaps the outstanding additional advantage of this unit is that the range of calf pens is portable and can be dismantled and sterilised at will.

The owner of this particular unit—who is, incidentally, also the manufacturer of the portable pens—keeps calves here from the age of 48 hours to six weeks. Then he dismantles and sterilises the pens, scrubs and disinfects the entire house and rests it (completely empty) for 14 days before stocking up again. *(Above.)*

The individual pens are big enough to allow the calves complete freedom of movement, and the rear portion is roofed over to further ensure the maintenance of a constant temperature. The floor is a portable slatted platform with narrow spaces between the slats for urine drainage. *(Below.)*

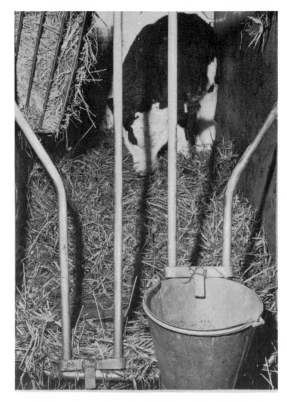

The final environmental advantage of this unit is that, though the calves are separated from one another, they still have a degree of communal living, because they can alleviate their boredom by seeing and licking the heads of their neighbours. (*Right.*)

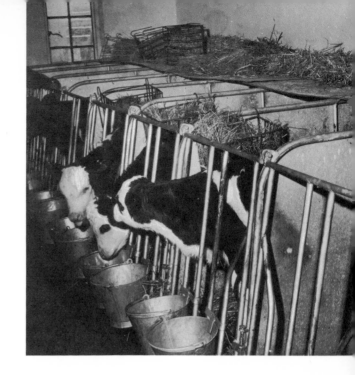

(c) Ideal environment by improvisation

A suitable environment for young calves can be created in any old or new building by the application of simple commonsense, bearing in mind the required conditions outlined in the introductory paragraph.

Briefly, the aim should be to create dry, insulated, draught-proof kennels within the main buildings.

This can be done anywhere by using straw bales, scrap wood, wire netting, sacks and loose straw, all of which are readily available on even the smallest holding. Add to this a nine-inch layer of ashes underneath the bedding and the young calves can be as constantly comfortable as in any air-conditioned building. (*Right.*)

Just two important points. The improvised false roof must be *complete* and must fit tightly against the back and side walls, otherwise it may attract draughts. And, secondly, there must be no cracks, crevices, or holes in the back or side walls. Only the front should be open and the size of the opening can be reduced or enlarged

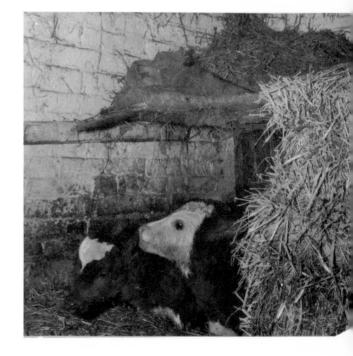

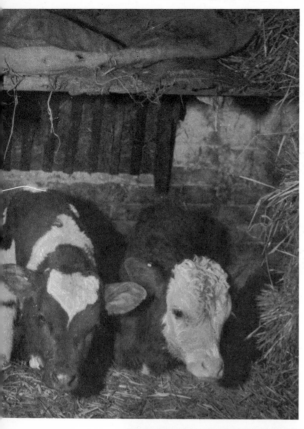

as required—again making use of the straw bales. *(Left.)*

A more permanent false roof can be provided by using timber beams to support the wire netting and straw but, again, to be fully effective, the roof has to be complete and fit tightly against the back and side walls. *(Below.)*

It is not necessary to cover over the entire pen if the outside structure is reasonably sound. Cover over at least three-quarters of the way from the back wall—i.e. make sure that, where the calves are lying during the night particularly, their body heat is being maintained as near constant as possible.

There are two ways you can tell whether the temperature is right—either by sitting in the pen for an hour on a cold night, or by installing maximum and minimum thermometers. But remember, provided the calves are healthy, it is not so important to get the temperature high as it is to maintain it at a *constant* level.

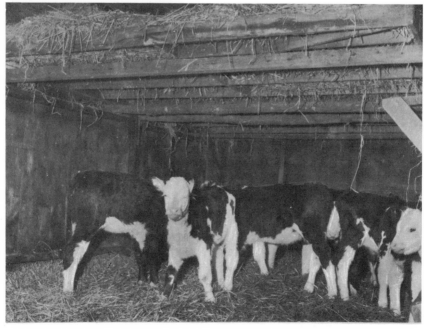

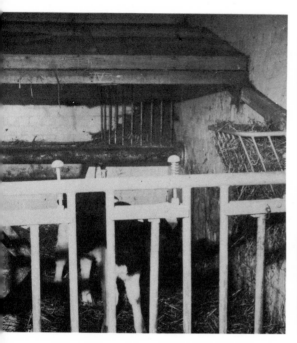

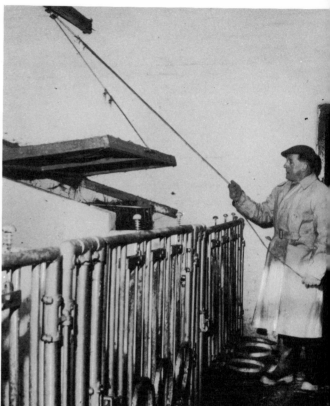

A slightly more elaborate but completely effective improvisation can be provided by a hinged, insulated, false roof which drops tightly into position to cover over three-quarters of the pen. The hinged portion can be turned back as and when the calves get over six weeks of age. *(Top, left and right.)*

The advantage here is that the individual kennels are comparatively small and compact. This allows the build-up and maintenance of a constant temperature, even though it only provides sufficient space for two or at the most three calves to be raised communally. Miniature hay rack, corn hopper and drinking bowl complete the compact amenities. Once again, the straw bedding is laid on a thick layer of loose ashes.

In some respects, a less permanent roof is preferable because it makes the biennial task of cleaning, disinfecting and resting somewhat easier.

(d) The hospital box

I am convinced that every stock farm in the world should have a hospital pen, or pens in which the stockman can nurse a weak or sickly calf. Daily on my rounds I see an appalling loss and wastage directly due to the lack of this simple facility.

A dry comfortable bed underneath, and the luxuriant warm radiance of an infra-red lamp above, can make all the difference between life or death to the calf which has been shocked by a protracted or difficult birth or by the toxins of a debilitating illness.

The Ideal Hospital Pen

The ideal layout is illustrated clearly in this plan and in the photographs. *(Below and right.)* The unit illustrated cost only £170 to build, including the internal galvanised framework. The pen should be sited facing south or south-west and should be well away from healthy calves or adult stock.

The best bedding to use for the sick calf is sawdust because, apart from its warmth

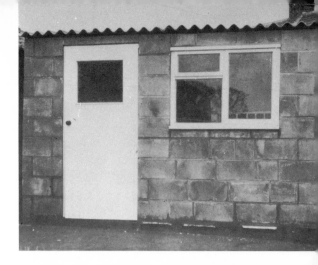

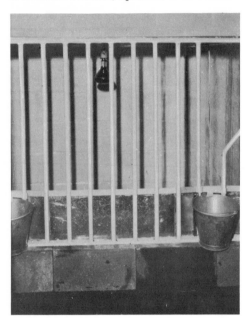

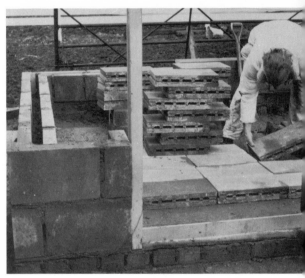

HOSPITAL PEN FOR CALVES

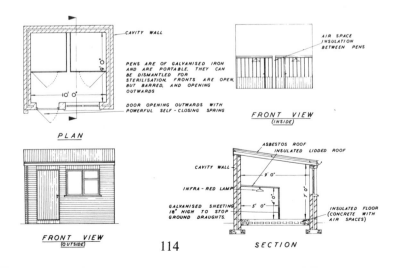

CAVITY WALL

PENS ARE OF GALVANISED IRON AND ARE PORTABLE. THEY CAN BE DISMANTLED FOR STERILISATION. FRONTS ARE OPEN, BUT BARRED, AND OPENING OUTWARDS

DOOR OPENING OUTWARDS WITH POWERFUL SELF-CLOSING SPRING

PLAN

AIR SPACE INSULATION BETWEEN PENS

FRONT VIEW
(INSIDE)

FRONT VIEW
(OUTSIDE)

ASBESTOS ROOF
INSULATED LIDDED ROOF

CAVITY WALL

INFRA-RED LAMP

GALVANISED SHEETING 18" HIGH TO STOP GROUND DRAUGHTS

INSULATED FLOOR (CONCRETE WITH AIR SPACES)

SECTION

114

and absorbent qualities, the sawdust makes the daily cleaning out very much easier.

The Improvised Hospital Pen

For the improvised unit, stick to the basic sizes recommended for the ideal pen. For the walls, make use of a corner and straw bales. For the roof, either wire netting or wood slats covered over with sacks and straw. For the floor, a foot of loose ashes underneath the bedding.

The infra-red lamp should be at least one foot to eighteen inches above the back of the calf when the calf is standing. *(Right.)*

Just one very important point, make absolutely certain that the improvised false roof fits tightly against the walls and on top of the bales.

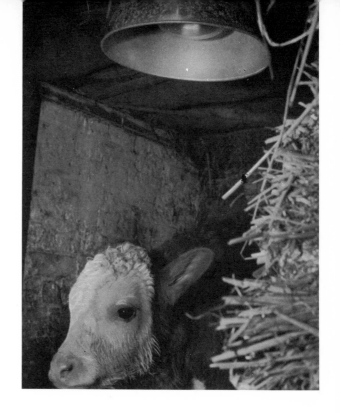

16
Rearing the Calf

DURING RECENT years calf losses have assumed fantastic proportions. One local knacker-man told me that in less than a week he collected over a thousand dead calves, and this is just one single knacker-yard. If you consider such losses on a national scale, they become frightening—almost epidemic—and the position continues to worsen.

I am convinced that the losses are due almost entirely to a complete disregard of the simple physiology of the calf's digestive system. The disregard is not intentional, but is largely due to the pressures of modern farming. But one thing is certain—the losses will continue unless every stock farmer takes careful heed of everything that is written here.

When a calf is born its fourth stomach—called the abomasum—is at least three times the size of its first stomach or rumen. *(Below, left.)* The reason for this is simply that Nature intends the calf to utilise its *fourth* stomach as its *main digestive organ* during the early part of its life.

When the calf starts sucking the cow—wagging its tail and perhaps bunting the udder but with its head held upwards, a groove called the 'oesophageal groove' at the bottom of the oesophagus or food pipe forms into a closed tube. *(Below, right.)*

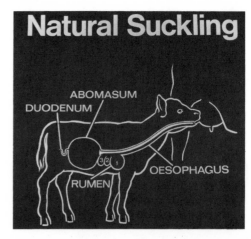

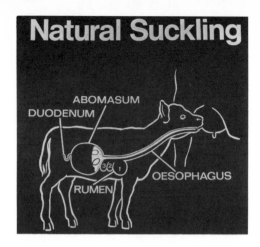

Natural Suckling

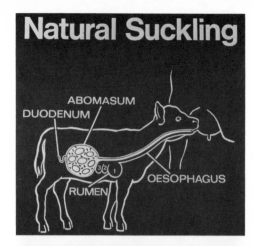

Natural Suckling

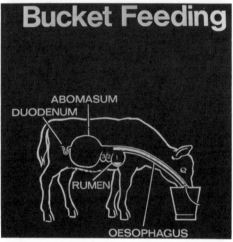

Bucket Feeding

The suckled milk then passes straight into the abomasum, bypassing the first, second and third stomachs. This is Nature's design for calf digestion.

In natural suckling the calf feeds frequently—approximately every two hours—and each time it does a clot forms in the abomasum. *(Above, left.)*

At the end of a day the abomasum contains a number of small clots, each one being acted on around the outside by the digestive juices. *(Above, right.)* There is *absolutely no space left* for any other type of foodstuffs and this is *exactly how Nature wants it to be.*

From two to three days onwards *ad lib* hay, corn and fresh clean water should always be provided. As the calf grows, he nibbles more and more of the hay and corn and drinks the correct amount of water. The hay, corn and water passes directly into the rumen or first stomach. Gradually this stomach develops and increases in size so that when the calf is ready for weaning towards the end of the eighth week, the position is reversed—the rumen is at least three times the size of the abomasum and is ready and able to take on the main task of ruminant digestion.

Bucket Feeding

When a calf is being suckled out of a bucket with its head down, the tube formation at the bottom of the oesophagus is not so complete and a fair percentage of the suckled milk filters off into the rumen or first stomach where it is virtually wasted. *(Above, right.)*

When the calf is being bucket-fed twice daily—as happens on most farms—only two clots are formed in the abomasum. *(Below.)* These are obviously not as big as they should be and certainly they don't by any means completely fill the stomach cavity. What happens then? Because of the comparatively long periods between the feeds, the calf gets hungry; it nibbles more than its quota of hay and corn and perhaps drinks an excess of water.

Bucket Feeding

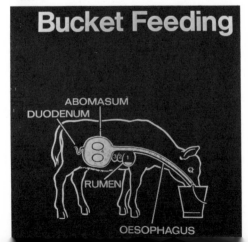

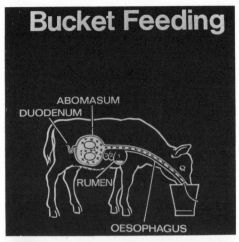

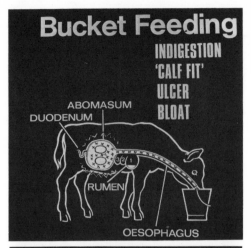

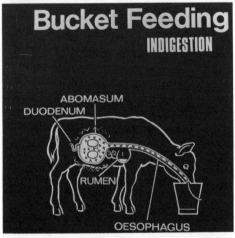

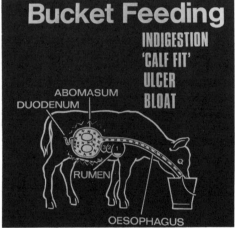

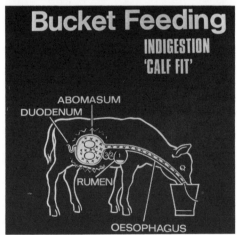

Some of the fibrous foods—undigested —find their way through into the empty spaces in the abomasum and when this happens the troubles really start. *(Top left.)*

The fibre irritates the inside lining of the abomasum and leads to indigestion. *(Second left.)*

The same irritation can produce the calf fit, which is often fatal. *((Third left.)*

Where the irritation is excessive, an ulcer may form; this in turn leads to bloat—another nuisance that can be fatal. *(Top right.)*

But, worst of all, the fibre may block up the very narrow exit from the abomasum into the duodenum. *(Second right.)* When this happens, the calf receives only a fraction of its available nourishment and literally starts to fade away suffering from every kind of protein, carbohydrate and vitamin deficiency until eventually it goes off its legs and dies.

At the same time, the lowered resistance caused by all these troubles leaves the calf an easy prey to scours and all the other killer diseases.

This, in my opinion, is the simple explanation of why so much money is lost in calf rearing. It is because the undigested fibre gets into the empty spaces in the abomasum, empty spaces that shouldn't be there. What action should be taken? Here's the drill I advise.

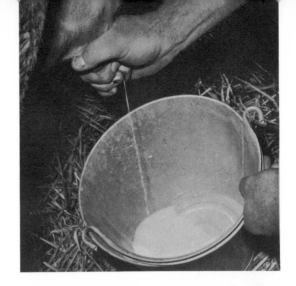

Drill to Follow

First of all, there is the matter of colostrum. The calf is capable of taking up its full quota of colostral antibodies *only when it is around four hours old*, so if you are lucky enough to see the calf born, milk off a pint of colostrum four hours later and drench the calf with it. *(Top right.)* Without the colostral antibodies the calf has no natural resistance against disease.

A better idea is to let the calf suck the mother for at least 24 hours, and the best idea of all is to rear the calf on the cow. *(Second right.)*

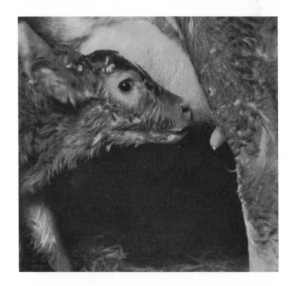

If you can't suckle your calves on cows, then use an artificial suckler, which ensures that the calf's head is held at the correct angle and that the oesophageal groove functions properly. Also, with the artificial suckler the calf keeps helping itself as it would do on a cow and the abomasum is kept full of small clots. *(Third right.)*

If you haven't got an artificial suckler, then for the first 14 days of the calf's life suckle it three times a day. This will mean three clots daily in the abomasum and will leave less room for the irritating fibre.

Use the mother's milk for the first week and bulk milk for the second, introducing the milk substitute only towards the end of that period.

Water is absolutely vital. Without water rumenal digestion cannot begin to take place because digestion in the rumen is a fermentative process. But the water must be clean and fresh. *(Following page.)*

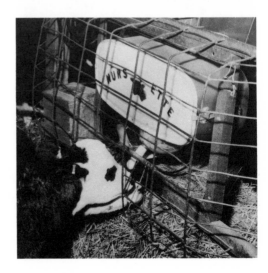

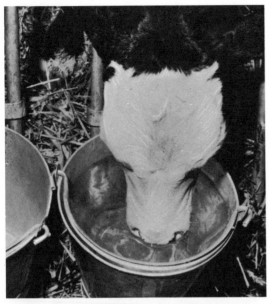

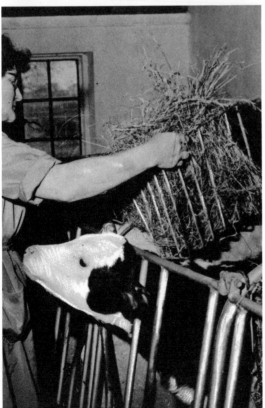

For fibrous food provide best quality hay fed at head level from the second or third day, and corn from the third or fourth day. *(Below, left.)*

If you do all this, then you can wean your calves suddenly, without any losses or troubles towards the end of the eighth week. At this age the calf's digestive system is fully developed and ready to cope with normal bovine food.

But remember; it's not much use developing perfect feeding techniques and then keeping the calves in draughty death-trap houses with soaking wet floors. Don't forget to give them draught-proof kennels and warm dry floors (see previous chapter).

To sum up. Get as close to Nature as you can and you'll stop your calf losses.

Feeding the Bought-in Calf

If the purchased calf looks in any way under the weather, it should be put in the hospital pen for a few days. If it is apparently healthy and vigorous, then it can go straight into the rearing pen.

For the first *two* liquid feeds, it should be given at each 5 lb of water (at blood heat) containing 4 tablespoonfuls of powdered glucose. Ad lib hay should be available, but no nuts or additional water. After 24 hours, put the calf straight onto milk or milk substitute, depending on its age or system of feeding, and introduce the nuts and ad lib water.

If this extremely simple routine is followed religiously, provided the calf pen floor and environment are up to scratch, losses and diseases should be kept to an absolute minimum.

17
Calf Scour

THERE ARE three common types of calf scour: the Digestive Type; the so-called White Scour or E. coli infection; and the dreaded Salmonella Scour.

(a) The digestive type

Cause

This occurs mainly when a calf is sucking on a cow which is giving too much milk. *(Right.)* The diarrhoea is due simply to an excess of milk, which passes straight through the stomachs into the calf's small intestine. Similar scour can be produced by bucket feeding to excess, but this is much less common.

A simple digestive scour occasionally arises as a result of too rapid changes in the diet, irregular feeding, or feeding too hot or too cold, but in such cases the picture is usually complicated by a flare up of E.coli infection.

Symptoms

Whenever you have scour occuring in a calf or calves that are sucking on a cow, then the condition is a simple digestive scour in ninety-nine cases out of a hundred. The faeces (dung) is usually yellow in colour.

Treatment

Take the calf off the cow for 24 hours. During that time give two feeds each of 5 lb of warm water containing 4 or 5

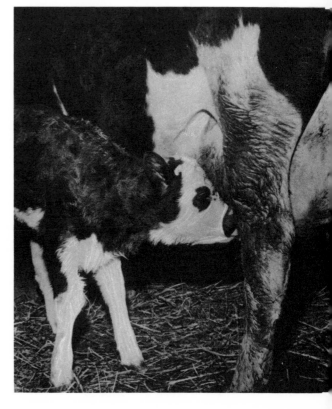

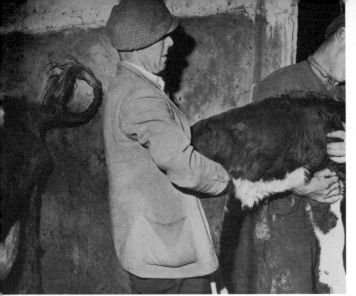

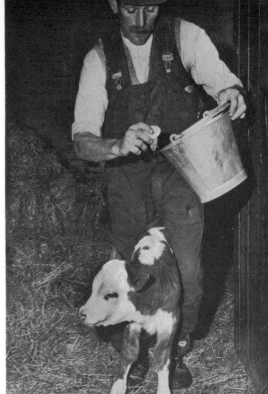

tablespoonfuls of powdered glucose and a switched-up raw egg. Thereafter, for the next three days, restrict the calf's sucking to three minutes three times a day. *(Above, left and right.)*

This simple treatment will cure the digestive scour most effectively. If, however, the scouring persists, it often indicates that bacterial complications have set in and it may be necessary to proceed with the routine prescribed for the E. coli scour.

Prevention

Obviously, it is unwise to put a single calf on a cow giving a lot of milk. The general rule I recommend is one calf per three-quarters of a gallon of the cow's estimated milk yield.

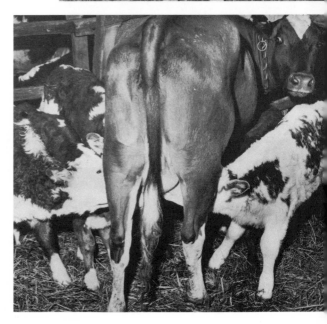

By their consistent sucking, the individual calves will stretch this estimated three-quarters to at least the full gallon. I know many successful calf rearers who allocate one sucking calf per half gallon—certainly it is better that the calf should have to work for its ration. *(Right.)*

In other words, the best way to prevent digestive scour in calves is to get back as near as possible to nature.

(b) White scour or E. coli infection

This is undoubtedly by far the most common type of scour encountered.

Cause

The specific cause is a germ called the E.coli, but there are a number of different types or strains of E.coli and these types may vary considerably in different countries and in different parts of any country. The germ is a normal resident of the

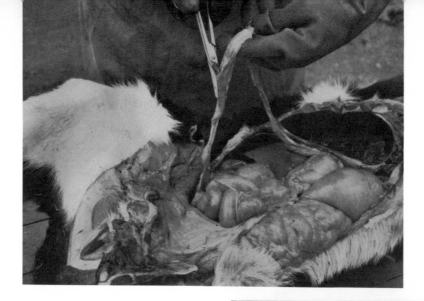

intestines of practically every calf, although the calf picks the germ up by the mouth after it is born. *(Above.)*

Predisposing Factors

Any factor which lowers the resistance of a calf can predispose to white scour by allowing the E.coli to multiply and grow strong. The common factors are:

1. Lack of colostrum, so that the calf has no antibodies and consequently no resistance against the E.coli.
2. Exposure to rapid changes in environmental temperature (see chapter on housing).
3. Cold, wet floors and bedding.
4. Transport to markets and exposure for long periods in the market pens. *(Right.)*
5. Irregular feeding, overfeeding, feeding at inconstant temperature.
6. Keeping calves continually in the same box. Here the germs increase in number and become progressively more dangerous.

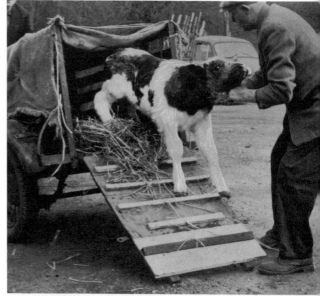

Symptoms

White diarrhoea associated with a fall in body temperature, while the calf's ears and tail become ice-cold to the touch.

Later, if untreated, the calf becomes prostrate, dehydrated and anaemic, the eyes become sunken and the inside of the mouth cold and clammy. When the calves reach this stage, they rarely respond to treatment. *(Right.)*

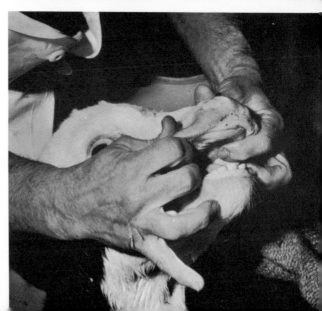

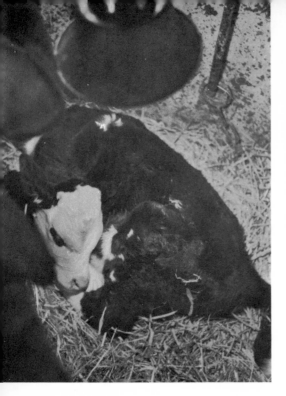

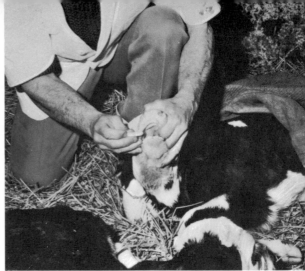

laboratory immediately. *(Below.)* There the E.coli can be identified and drug sensitivity tests can be done inside twenty-four hours. This allows the veterinary surgeon to apply the most effective specific treatment.

4. Pending this laboratory investigation, a general broad spectrum antibiotic combined with a bowel sulpha drug should be given by the mouth. *(Above, right.)*

5. Vitamin injections, iron tonics and intravenous saline injections can also be used but these should be prescribed and given only by the veterinary surgeon.

Prevention

The obvious answer is to eliminate, so far as possible, the predisposing causes. Therefore, the routine should be:

1. Make certain the calves get their own

Treatment

1. Constant warmth is the first essential, so the patient should be immediately put under an infra-red lamp in a hospital pen, improvised or otherwise—see section on 'the hospital box'. *This is the most vital and important part of all scour treatment. (Above, left.)*

2. Milk or milk substitute should be witheld for 24 hours and warm water, raw egg and glucose used, as in digestive scour.

3. Swabs of faeces should be taken by your veterinary surgeon and sent to a

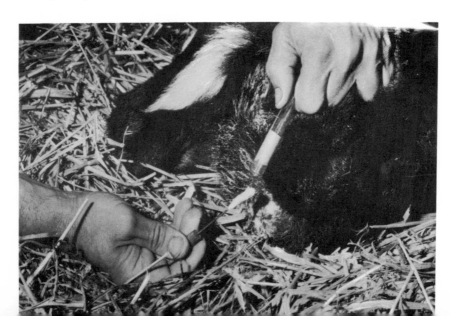

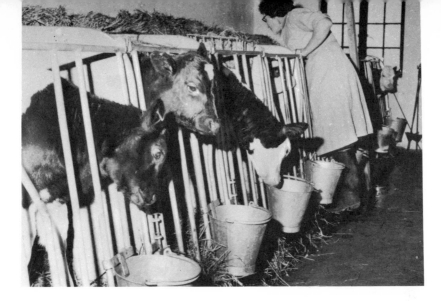

mother's colostrum or first milk for at least the first five days of life, but especially in the period from 24 to 48 hours after birth.

2. Get the floors, housing and environment to the standards specified in the previous chapters, going all out for a constant temperature and a dry floor. (*Above.*)

3. Avoid buying from markets if possible.

4. Pay special attention to regular and correct transistional feeding as recommended in the chapter on feeding the calf.

5. Every three months, empty the calf pens completely. Scrub with hot water, soda and disinfectant and leave completely empty for at least fourteen days. This will eliminate the risk of disease build-up.

Do all this and you will get little, if any, scour or losses in calves. Don't do all this and you deserve all the trouble and deaths you will most certainly encounter.

(c) The Salmonella scour

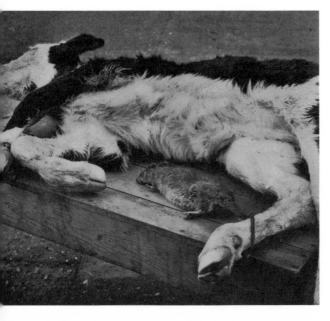

Cause

Chiefly a germ called the Salmonella dublin, although another member of the same group—the Salmonella typhimurium—can also cause a great deal of trouble.

There are five sources:

(a) Infected calves

(b) Recovered cows

(c) Pigs, poultry and human beings which can be infected by Salmonella typhimurium

(d) The infection can persist in rats (*Left.*)

(e) Infected buildings, transport vehicles, and markets

The Salmonella germ can live in a dirty building for several years.

How it Spreads

Just one single infected calf from a market, a transport vehicle or from a dealer's premises, is all that is necessary to create havoc. In other words, Salmonellosis is a disease which is spread chiefly by bought-in calves. *(Right.)*

Fortunately, the recovered 'carrier' cow is a rarity because Salmonellosis is usually fatal in adult cattle. But Salmonella typhi-murium infection can frequently flare up in pigs and poultry and the germ can be carried to the calves via the feet and clothing of the attendants.

Nowadays, human infection is also comparitively rare.

Salmonella, once introduced, can affect the healthiest of calves but, nonetheless, the poorer the management the more likely the infection is to persist and gain strength. Thoughtless and improper feeding, cold and draughty pens, wet or inadequate bedding—one of these can lower the calf's resistance to such an extent that it stands little chance of survival

If you add to that periods of starvation in cold, draughty markets and the jolting transport journeys, it is easy to understand why Salmonellosis can become an endemic problem.

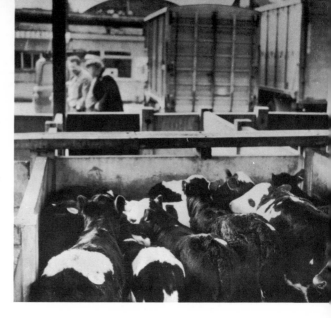

Where it Differs

It appears to attack chiefly the older calves—calves three, four or up to six weeks of age—at an age beyond the usual calf scour period though, of course, young calves are also highly susceptible. The average calf receives, in the colostrum, antibodies against E.coli scour but only rarely against Salmonella. Consequently, when Salmonella is introduced the results can be disastrous, with a death rate of up to 50 per cent. *(Below.)*

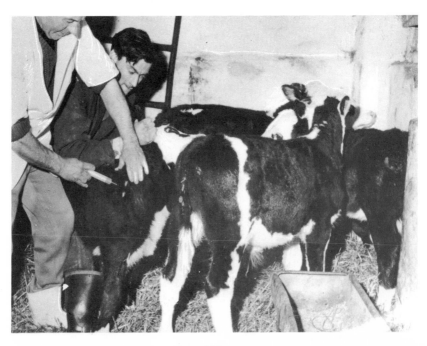

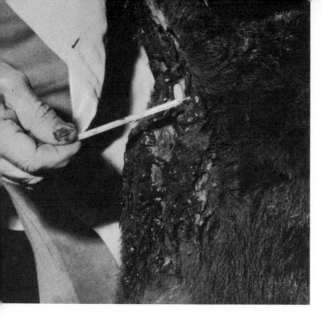

Symptoms
The germs cause an inflammation of the stomach and intestines, and give rise in calves to an elevated temperature (around 105°), with a diarrhoea varying from yellow to dark coloured and bloodstained, depending on the degree of severity. *(Above.)*

The illness runs a course of five to six days, but in hyperacute cases the calves may die in from 24 to 72 hours, sometimes with little or no signs of scour. Occasion-ally the picture is complicated by the development of a well-marked pneumonia.

Treatment
A veterinary surgeon should be called in immediately. He will take swabs of the faeces and will culture and identify the germ in a laboratory. *(Below.)*

Mortality is about 50 per cent, despite the wide range of drugs at our disposal. It is my experience that only furazolidone and terramycin appear in any way effective, and even these need the help of vitamin injections and simple old-fashioned reme-dies like kaolin, chalk, stout, eggs and brandy.

Obviously, therefore, with Salmonella, it is much better to concentrate on prevention.

Prevention
A Salomonella vaccine is now available and this should go a long way to reducing the incidence. However, to be completely effective, the vaccine use must be combined

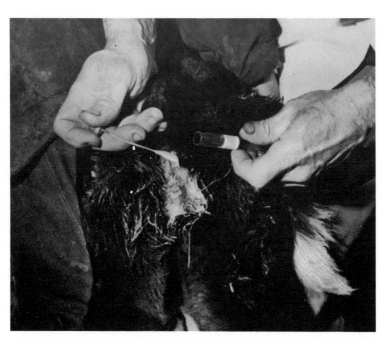

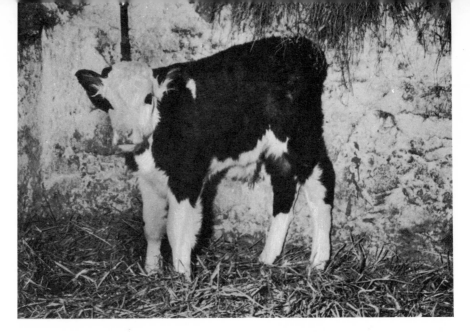

with commonsense husbandry, if only because the vaccine takes fourteen days to produce its protection.

If you've had the infection, clean the box out very thoroughly with hot water and soda, disinfect, and leave empty for at least fourteen days before restocking with vaccinated calves. At the same time, organise an all-out attack on the rat population.

If you haven't had the infection, aim at keeping the herd self-contained. If unable to do this and you have to buy, watch your management carefully.

First, if possible, purchase from known disease-free sources. I know farmers who travel hundreds of miles to collect calves simply to make sure of their origin.

Second, don't mix new calves with residents for at least 14 days. *(Above.)*

Third, make sure your calf pens are clean, dry, warm and draught proof—see chapter on housing.

And, last, watch the feeding very carefully during the settling-in period—see chapter on feeding the calf. Any stomach or bowel upset can lower the calf's resistance and allow the bug to gain hold. It is often during the transition period of dietetical change that disease flares up.

I cannot emphasise too strongly that the better the calf's condition, feeding and environment, the less likely it is to succomb to any disease.

18
Calf Diphtheria

CALF DIPHTHERIA is a simple condition which, in my experience, is little understood by the average farmer or stockman. It is a common disease occurring everywhere and is one of the easiest of all calf diseases to diagnose and treat.

Cause

Calf diphtheria is caused by the same germ that causes foul in the foot—the Fusiformis necròphorus.

The Fusiformis necrophorus is a normal resident of the feet of a high percentage of cattle, living in the cracks between the wall and the sole. *(Right.)* It can live in the dung and in the bedding, but only for about a month at the most. Whilst outside, it can live on the pasture for a maximum of fourteen days.

The germ gets into the calf's mouth simply through the calf eating contaminated bedding or contaminated fodder. It gets a hold through wounds, scratches or cuts in the linings of the mouth cavity. The scratches can be caused by straw, barley piles, thistles or thorns.

As soon as the germ gains entrance into

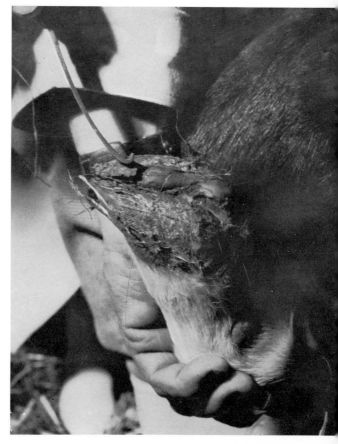

the wound, it multiplies and grows and produces a lump of dead tissue, in exactly the same way as it does in a case of foul. (*Right.*)

How To Spot It

During the multiplication of the germ, the affected part of the jaw becomes painful and the calf shows a disinclination to eat or take its suckling. The temperature is usually normal but the patient is dull and listless and is not keen to stand or move around.

Later on, the only symptom is a lump on the side of the jaw and, in the majority of cases, this is the first symptom seen. (*Below.*)

Occasionally, the germ attacks the soft tissues of the tongue and the back of the

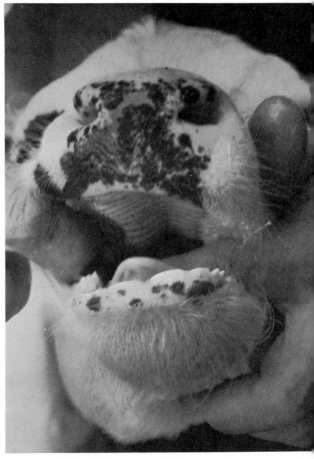

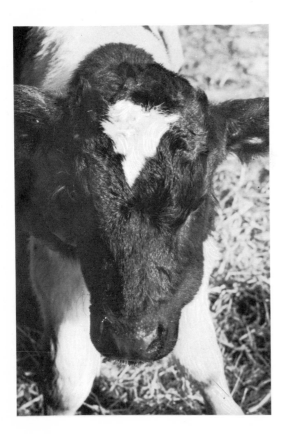

throat. When this happens, the outstanding symptom is an inability to swallow—boluses of partially chewed hay are found in the back of the mouth and the calf's breath smells like dead meat. Naturally, condition is rapidly lost.

What To Do

Fortunately, nowadays treatment presents no problem, provided it is started in reasonable time. As in the case of foul, all the sulpha drugs and antibiotics are virtually specific. When the sulpha drugs

130

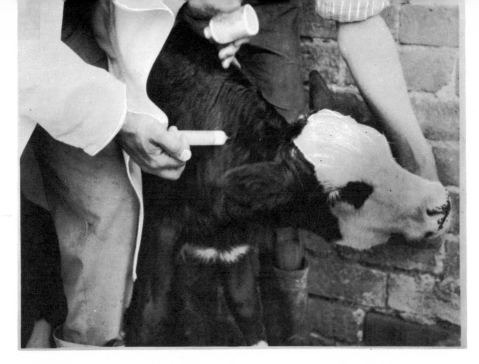

or antibiotics are given by injection, then two doses will usually suffice. When given by the mouth, a four or five-day course is required. *(Above and below.)*

How To Prevent It

There is no vaccine against the Fusiformis and, therefore, once again the best means of defence lies in cleanliness and good husbandry.

In the first place, calves should be housed in a box which has been cleaned,

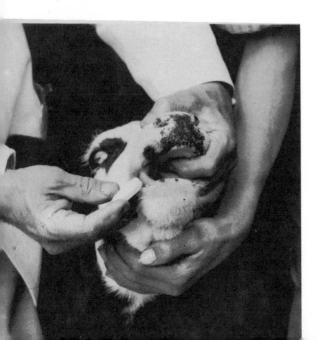

disinfected and rested for at least one month before their entry.

Water ad lib should be provided from birth and ample hay should always be fed from a rack or net. It is my experience that calves will rarely if ever eat straw when good hay is available.

Wet bedding seems to favour the persistence of the germ and, therefore, the floor underneath the straw should be insulated and well drained or, if not, it should be covered by a good thick layer of ashes.

Where the disease is a special problem, it may be a good plan to scrape the cracks in the calves' feet thoroughly with a black-smith's knife and afterwards to soak them individually in a 10% solution of formalin, or some other mild antiseptic.

Many people say that calf diphtheria is only found where the husbandry is bad. I wouldn't go the length of saying this, but I would say that it is much less likely to occur where the husbandry is good. It is not a fatal condition, but it is a disease which every good stockman should know about.

19
Joint-Ill

JOINT-ILL usually affects young calves round about a week or ten days old although occasionally the symptoms may appear at three weeks or even a month. *(Below, right.)*

Cause

Joint-ill in calves may be caused by a variety of germs, the commonest being the simple streptococcus which can be present almost anywhere.

In a pen where calves are continually housed, the germs appear to get progressively more dangerous because the number of cases will increase—this goes also for other germs which cause scour and pneumonia. In other words, there occurs a disease build-up. *(Below, left.)*

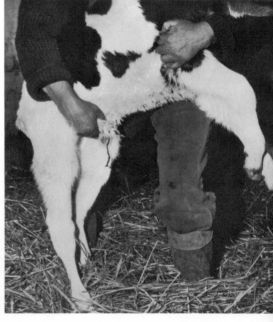

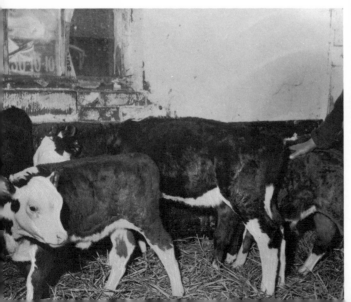

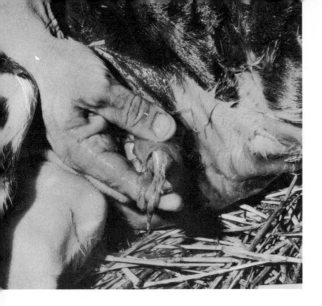

Symptoms

The affected calf or calves—often there is more than one affected—start to walk stiffly. At the same time they go off their feed and run a high temperature of 105° or 106°. The navel is usually swollen and there may be a painful puffiness in one or several of the joints. *(Below, left.)*

In long-standing cases, abscesses form in the joints and these may burst externally. *(Below, right.)*

Entrance and Effect

The joint-ill bugs can gain entry through an abrasion or wound but usually they get in via the calf's navel during the first two or three days of life. *(Above.)* Just occasionally, joint-ill can flare up as a complication of some other debilitating disease.

The germs get into the bloodstream and are carried to the various joints where they multiply and produce inflammation and swelling, and eventually pus if allowed to progress without treatment.

Treatment

Fortunately, the sulpha drugs and the complete range of antibiotics are specific against the common types of joint-ill. But

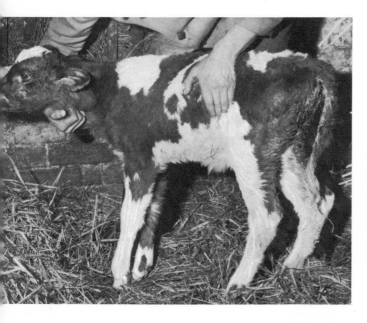

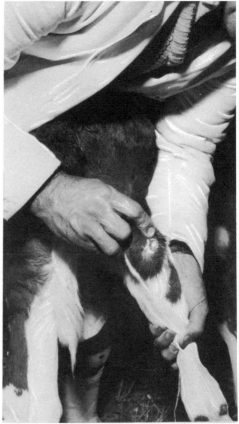

the drugs should be used carefully and only under veterinary supervision. *(Right.)*

Prevention

Scrub, disinfect and rest the calving boxes for 14 days at least twice a year; and scrub, disinfect and rest the calf pens at least four times a year. This breaks the cycle of the disease build-up. *(Below, left.)*

Use plenty of clean bedding in the calving box during and after each calving, and subsequently in the calf pens when the calves are transferred there.

Dress the navel of the new-born calf with an antiseptic or antibiotic dressing three times on the first and second day and twice on the third day of life. This precaution is especially important when the calves are taken from the mother at birth. *(Below, right.)*

An aerosol containing a powerful antibiotic and dye is ideal for this purpose, though sulpha powder dressings can be used, and even the old-fashioned painting

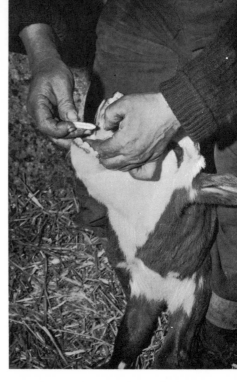

with tincture of iodine is a great deal better than nothing.

Lastly, and perhaps the most important point of all, the new or recently born calf should be put in a pen with a clean dry

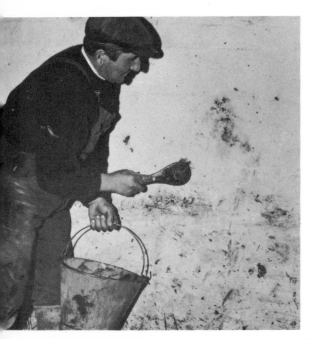

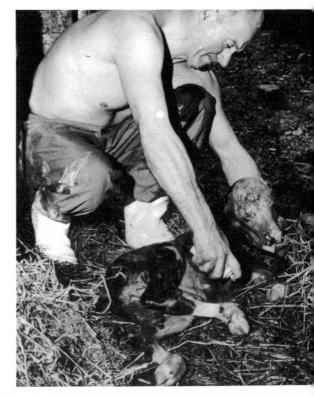

floor—see chapter on housing. The ideal is illustrated here—a single pen with a fitted sterilised slatted floor (narrow spaces between the slats) and lashings of clean straw. *(Right.)*

If ideal single pens are not available, then be certain to provide a thick layer of ashes underneath the straw bedding, floor spaces for urine drainage, or, at the very least, a good thick bed of clean sawdust.

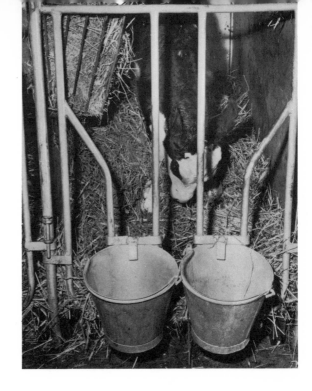

20
White Muscle Disease

THE CAUSE of this disease is a deficiency of vitamin E.
All normal farm rations contain ample amounts of vitamin E and the deficiency, therefore, occurs only under certain circumstances. For example, if the dams have been poorly fed and the calves have been reared on skim milk without access to good hay. Another possible cause is the feeding of excess cod-liver oil.

How to Recognise   *(Below, left.)*
The first symptom in the calf is sleepiness combined with an unwillingness to stand. When made to stand, the calf adopts unnatural postures and day by day the muscles around the top of the hind and fore-legs and in the rest of the skeleton waste away rapidly. *(Right.)* If the calf is untreated, it may finally become completely prostrated, show distressed abdom-

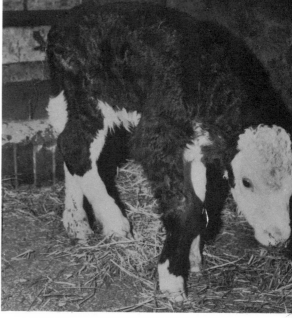

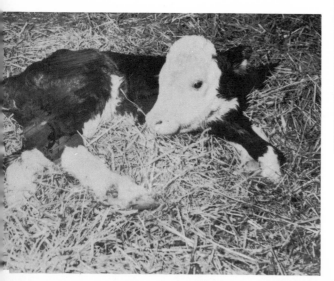

inal breathing, and die within a few days. If the calf is excited, it may fall down with a heart-attack.

136

How to Treat

It is important to start treatment at the earliest possible stage—if the condition becomes advanced, there is no cure.

As soon as the muscular weakness and degeneration is suspected, vitamin E in the form of tablets or in the form of wheat germ oil should be fed in small quantities daily in the suckling. Concentrated vitamin E injections can be given but I have found the daily small oral doses much more satisfactory. *(Above.)*

Combined with this medicinal treatment, ample good quality hay should be provided for the calf and, if possible, milk should be used for suckling. In other words, during the treatment period at least, milk substitutes should be avoided. If cod-liver oil is being fed, it should be stopped immediately.

How to Prevent

Prevention here is simple. It is merely a matter of good management and correct feeding.

The dam should be well fed, particularly during the latter half of pregnancy and should, in particular, have an ample supply of good hay or silage. Where the disease appears in silage-fed animals, then hay should be added to the dam's diet during the last two months of pregnancy. Cod-liver oil should not be fed, except under veterinary supervision.

Small amounts of wheat germ oil (approximately half a teaspoonful) can be fed daily for fourteen days. This is an effective but expensive preventative and is not usually necessary. *(Right.)*

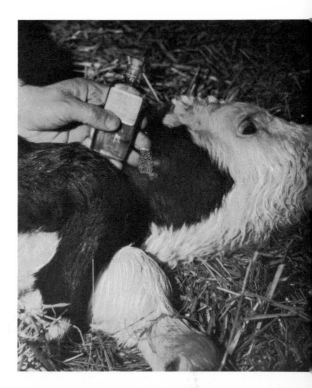

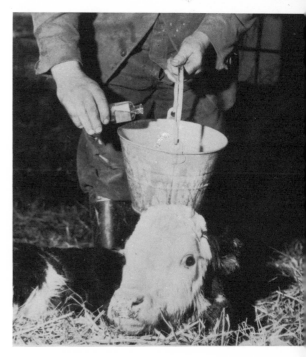

21
Vitamin A Deficiency

VITAMIN A is the essential growth vitamin. Without it, there is first of all a retardation and then a cessation of growth in all the body bones, muscles and tissues.

Normal Sources

Vitamin A is stored in the calf's liver. The chief natural sources to the young calf are first of all the mother's milk and later the bulk feed of hay, silage or haylage. The other usual source is provided by the vitamin-supplemented proprietary calf-rearing foodstuffs. *(Right.)*

Causes of Deficiency

Vitamin A deficiency is most likely to arise in weaned calves, under .normal circumstances, if they are being fed poor quality fibre and unsupplemented home-grown cereals. *(Top of next page.)*

   Excess feeding of barley when little or no hay is provided can precipitate severe attacks. Here the condition is produced, at least in part, by the widespread liver damage that so often occurs in intensive barley feeding.

Symptoms

General unthriftiness and failure or cessation of growth. The simple reason for this is because, as mentioned in the introduction, vitamin A is the growth vitamin and, when it is deficient or absent, all growth is correspondingly affected. The

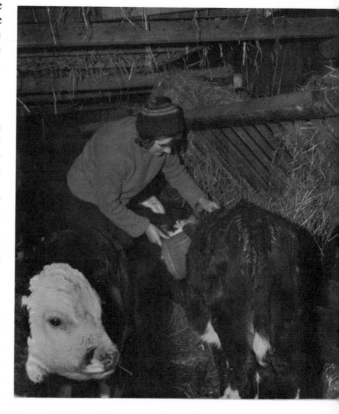

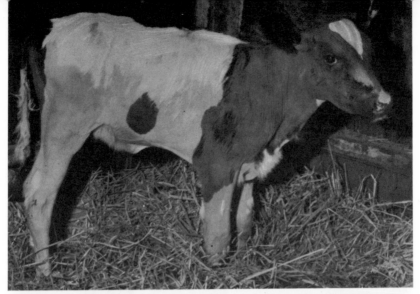

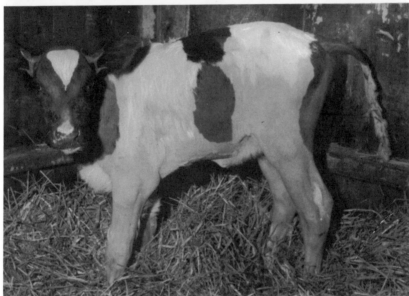

hair falls out and later the calf may stagger slightly when it moves. *(Above.)*

There occurs a thickening of the skin and, later, partial or complete blindness, with the eyes occasionally discharging. *(Right.)*

Treatment

If blindness is a symptom, it is usually permanent and it is best to slaughter the calf and concentrate on preventing symptoms appearing in the others. If the patient happens to be a bull calf being reared for breeding, then he should be slaughtered or castrated since his fertility is likely to be permanently damaged.

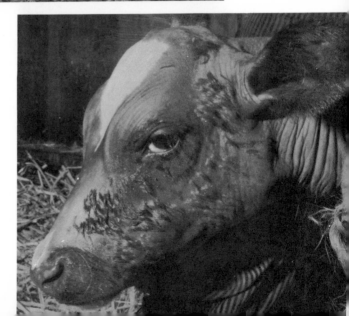

In addition to providing a natural or supplemented vitamin A source, 250 to 500 thousand international units of concentrated vitamin A should be injected intramuscularly into all the remaining calves. *(Right.)* Recovery will not be spectacular—it will be slow but progressive.

Prevention

The simple prevention, apart from sticking as closely as possible to traditional rearing methods, is to provide *ad lib* top-quality early-cut hay or high-quality silage or haylage. In intensive barley beef production the good quality fibre may be rationed, but a percentage is nonetheless essential. *(Below.)*

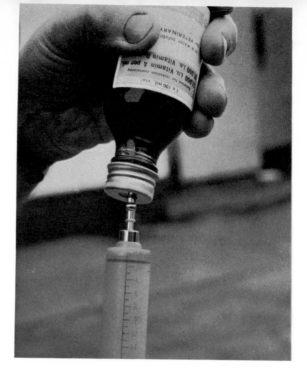

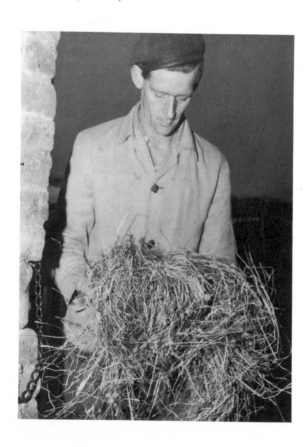

22
Contracted Tendons

TEN MILLION pounds worth of calves are being lost each year from thoughtlessness, carelessness, neglect and disease. This we are well aware of and are doing everything possible to remedy.

Just occasionally, however, the odd calf is scrapped because of an apparent deformity. One such case is the calf born with one or both fore legs bent forward as in the picture. *(Below, right.)* When it stands the fetlocks and/or the knees knuckle forward.

It is wrong to slaughter such calves because the vast majority will get better by themselves within the first two months of life.
The condition is due to a contraction of the flexor tendons which run down from the back of the knee joints to the bulbs of the heels. *(Below, left.)*

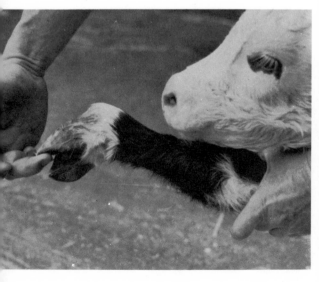

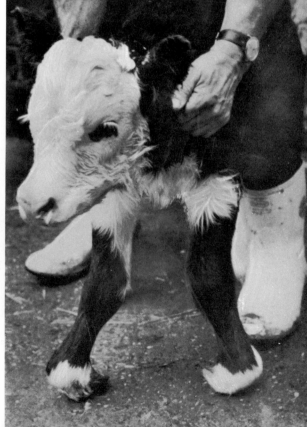

141

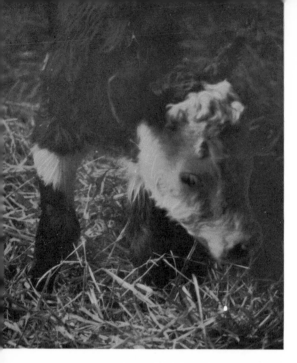

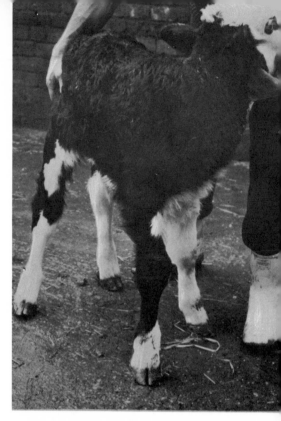

Even though, in the beginning, it seems difficult or impossible to straighten the affected leg, nature appears to relax the tendons gradually. One important point, however, when the calf is born with the legs straight and the contraction develops subsequently, the condition is much more serious and rarely, if ever, gets better. *(Below.)*

The only treatment required is to keep the calf on a deep, soft bed of built-up muck topped with straw. *(Above, left.)* If this is not done, the front of the fetlock joints may become lacerated or even worn through to the bone.

Just a few days of patience and care and the result is a healthy straight-legged calf growing into money. *(Above, right.)*

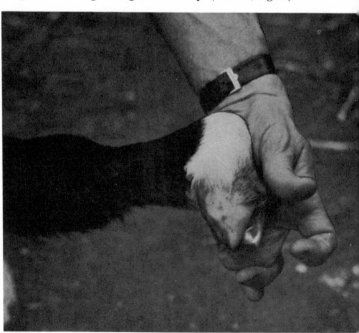

23
Dehorning

THE DEHORNING of calves is a task which can be done by any efficient farmer or stockman, but it is essential that the correct technique be employed. According to the law an anaesthetic must be used. General anaesthesia is dangerous and out of the reach of the farmer, but local anaesthesia is simple and most veterinary surgeons will be only too happy to instruct their clients in its use.

The calves should be done when under one month old. Usually around two weeks is the best age because by then the horn bud, though easily distinguishable, is not too well-developed. *(Below.)*

The Dehorner
All caustic preparations are dangerous and unreliable. The job should always be done with a correctly heated dehorning iron.

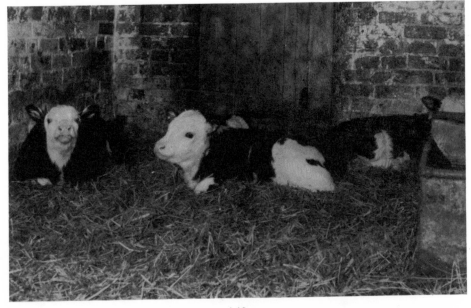

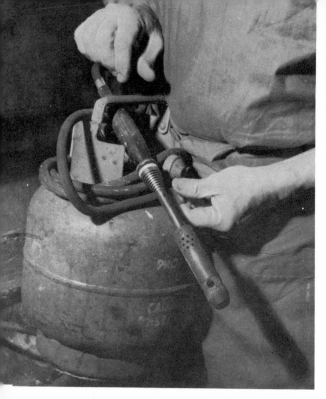

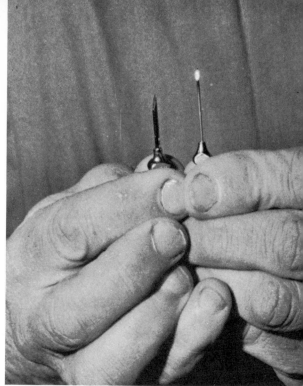

Electrically-heated dehorning irons are excellent but I have found that the most satisfactory all-purpose instrument is the one heated by calor gas, because calves are often kept in boxes where there is no electricity supply. The calor gas dehorner is efficient, easily transported and comparatively inexpensive. *(Above, left.)*

Other Tools Required

Local anaesthetic, syringe and needle, scissors, antiseptic and cotton wool. *(Below.)*

A number '18' needle about $\frac{3}{4}''$ long, i.e. the one on the right *(above)*, is ideal, although one with a shorter and thicker bore can be used provided the point is sharp. The needle should be at least $\frac{1}{2}''$ long because, in calves, the nerve to be blocked lies fairly deep at the site of injection.

An ordinary record syringe is ideal and

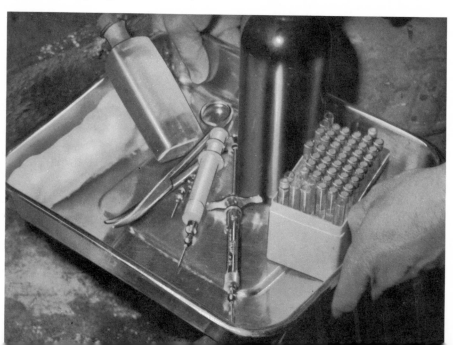

local anaesthetic can be supplied in bulk. *(Top, right.)*

A special cartridge-loading syringe can be bought which, though expensive, is perhaps more economical in the long run. The local anaesthetic is supplied in cartridges and one cartridge contains sufficient to anaesthetise two horn buds. *(Bottom, right.)*

The job can be done comfortably with the calf on its legs and its hind quarters in a corner. *(Below.)*

One or two assistants can keep the hind end in position, though one person is enough—in fact, the job can be done single-handed if necessary. The operator should

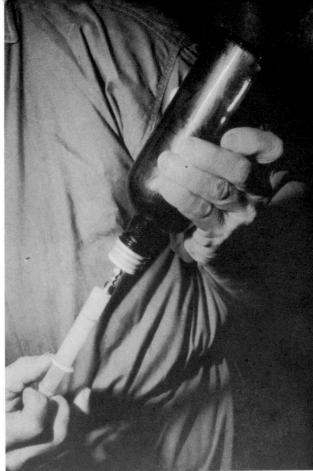

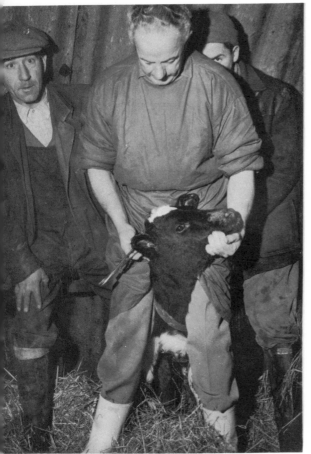

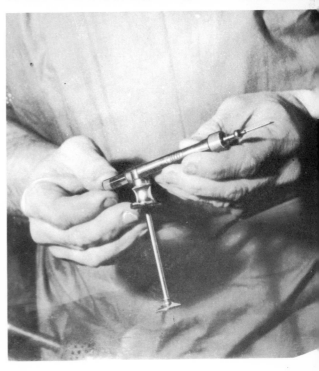

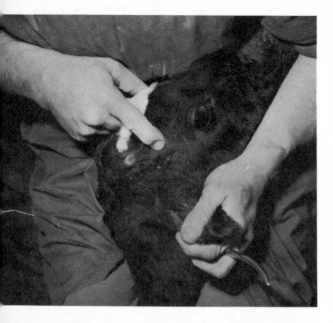

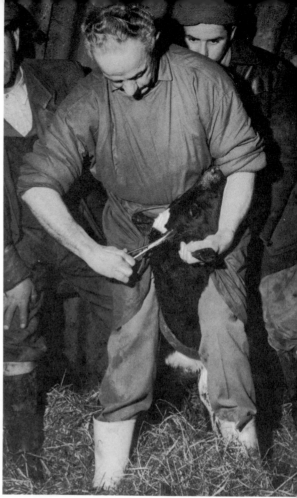

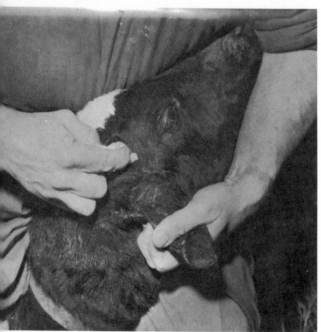

stand astride the shoulders of the calf, holding it firmly between his knees.

Technique

Dealing with the right horn bud, the operator should grasp the right ear with his left hand and tuck the nose of the calf along his left forearm. With the scissors he should now clip the hair over the horn and over the site of the injection. *(Above.)*

The site for injection of the anaesthetic is a spot about mid-way between the eye and the horn bud, and immediately below the ridge of bone which runs between these two.

The site should feel soft and pliable under the finger. *(Top, left.)*

After clipping the hair, the site should be coated with a powerful skin antiseptic. *(Bottom, left.)*

146

The Injection

The needle should be inserted fairly deeply and at right angles to the ridge. One c.c. (i.e. half a cartridge) of the local anaesthetic should be injected. *(Right.)*

One sure way of telling whether the needle is in the correct spot is by the ease with which the anaesthetic goes in. If the syringe plunger has to be forced, the needle should be withdrawn and inserted again slightly lower down.

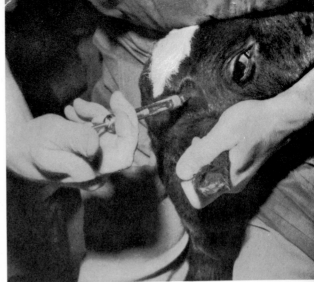

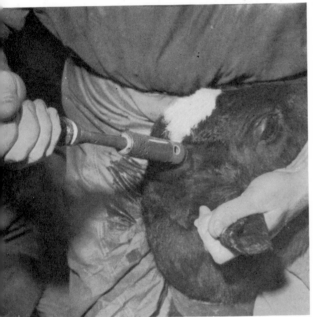

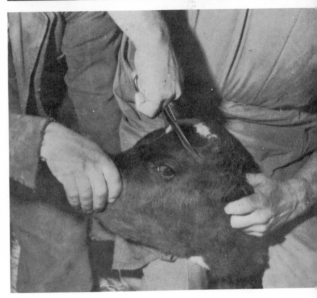

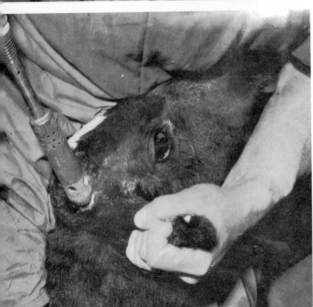

The clipping, disinfecting and injecting should now be repeated on the left side, this time the calf's head being held firmly against the right thigh of the operator by the right hand of the assistant. *(Above.)*

The Dehorning

The end of the dehorning iron should be placed over the bud and turned in a half circle ten or twelve times. *(Top, left.)*

The horn bud should now be 'dug out' by pressing the upper edge of the iron firmly inwards and downwards. *(Bottom, left.)*

It takes approximately five minutes for the anaesthetic to take full effect, an effect

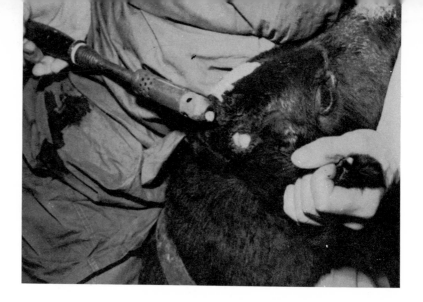

which lasts for at least one hour, so it's a good idea to anaesthetise all the calves that require dehorning before commencing the actual operation.

Evidence that the job is done correctly, and that the horn will never grown again, is the horn bud in the end of the dehorning iron and a clear hollow in the skin of the head where the bud has been. *(Above.)*

The left horn bud is now removed in exactly the same way. *(Below.)*

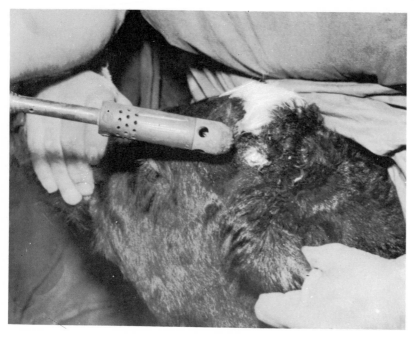

24
Removal of Accessory Teats

I'VE SEEN many honest attempts by herdsmen to remove accessory teats in calves but rarely, if ever, have I come across a perfect job.

The most common mistake is for the teat to be cut off level with, or even slightly below, the surrounding skin. This leaves a lump or a scar which gets more and more unsightly as the heifer grows. And if the amputation is attempted when the heifer is older, a milk fistula may result—i.e. a permanent hole which will leak milk after the heifer has calved.

There is, however, a simple technique which always ensures a first-class job.

First of all, get an assistant to turn the calf up and sit it on its hind end. Obviously, for easy handling, the younger the calf the better—I think it should be under two months old. *(Below.)*

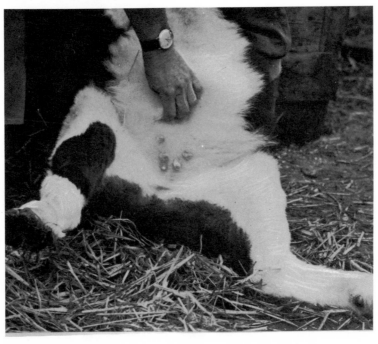

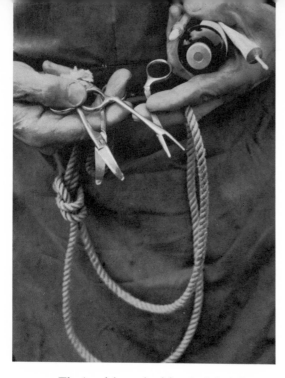

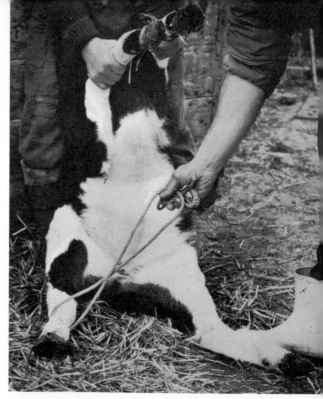

The 'tools' required for the job *(Above.)* are a looped cord; a pair of sharp curved surgical scissors; a pair of artery forceps; a small syringe; some local anaesthetic; and a tube of antibiotic. All these your veterinary surgeon can provide.

Take the rope, pass one side of the loop over the foot to just above the fetlocks, and twist it into a 'figure of eight.' *(Top, right.)*

Put the other side of the 'eight' over the other foot, and again up to just above the fetlock. *(Bottom, right.)*

Fix the calf's hind legs by placing one foot on the centre of the 'figure of eight'. This will save many a painful kick on the shins. *(Below.)*

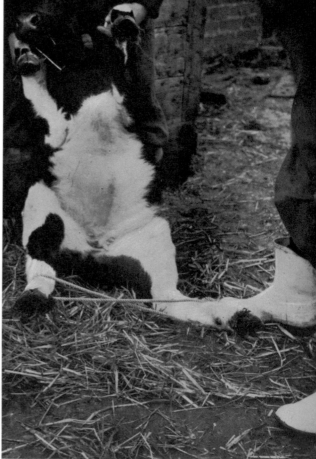

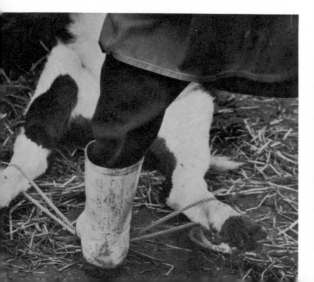

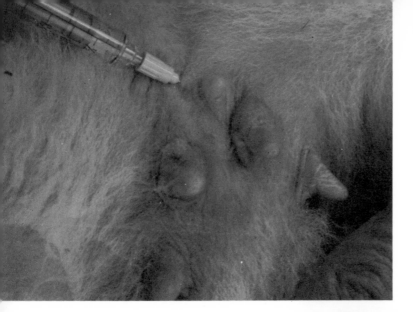

Insert half a c.c. of local anaesthetic underneath the skin at the base of the extra teat and leave for at least a minute. *(Above.)*

Grasp and fix the teat firmly in the jaws of the artery forceps. *(Right.)*

With the artery forceps, pull the teat outwards as far as possible, and then take a generous 'bite' with the curved scissors around the teat base. Don't be afraid to take a good portion of the surrounding skin. *(Below.)*

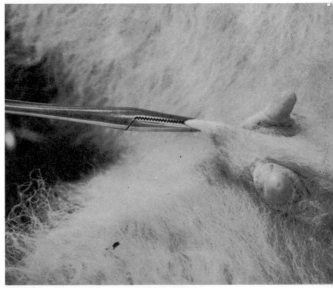

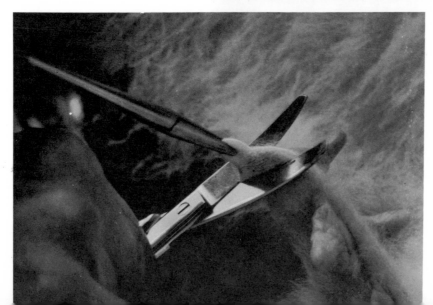

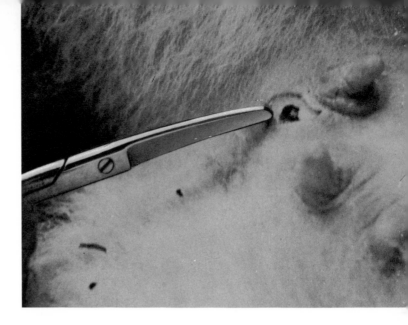

This leaves a comparatively large elliptical wound, but it ensures the complete removal of the rudimentary milk sinus which, if left, would produce the subsequent leaking. *(Above.)*

Finally, dress the wound thoroughly with the antibiotic. Any infection in this area, even in a young calf, can ruin the potential milk production. *(Below.)*

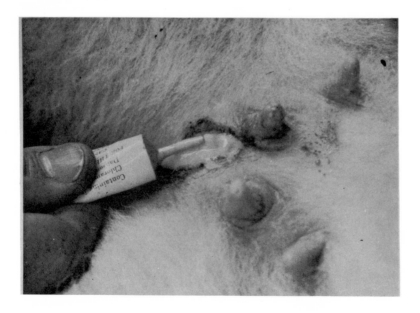

25
Lead Poisoning

ALL CATTLE, especially calves, are highly susceptible to poisoning by lead. A comparatively small quantity is enough to kill a calf and many of the mysterious outbreaks of illness and death among groups of stock in various parts of the country have eventually been traced to lead poisoning.

Where the Lead Comes From
The most common sources are *paint* and *roofing felt*. In fact, all the cases which I personally have had to investigate have been due to the animals licking or eating one or the other. *(Top of next page.)*

The felt, in itself, does not contain lead but it is often impregnated with lead paint. Felt may flake from the layer underneath

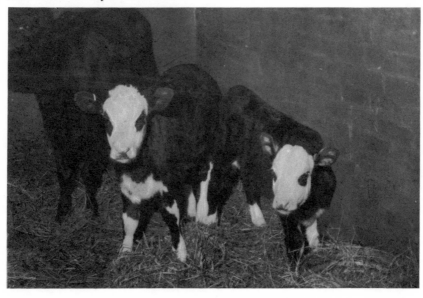

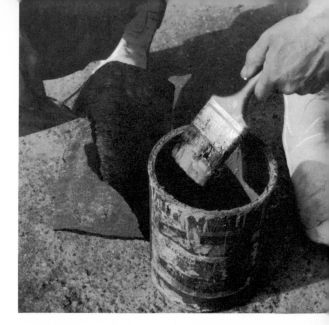

the tiles and fall onto the food, or it may have been used to patch up holes in walls or windows and attract the calves during their idle exploratory licking. (*Centre, right.*)

In most of the felt cases I have seen, portions—usually from old fowl pens—have been left lying about in the rick yard and have found their way into the boxes either in the bedding or in the hay. (*Below.*)

Many modern paints do not contain lead, but all the older paints did have lead in them and the basic paint work inside most of the older farmsteads comprises a great potential danger.

Only a few flakes of this old paint are required to produce symptoms in calves and yet, in many cases, calves have been reared without loss year after year in the same boxes with the identical paint on the doors. (*Bottom, right.*) This is simply be-

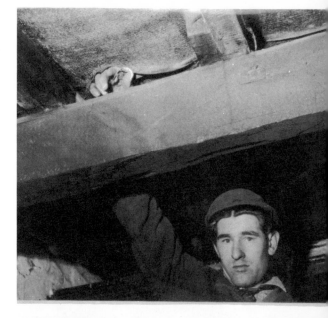

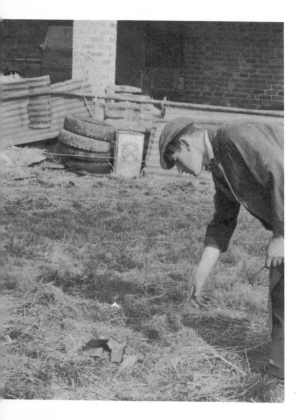

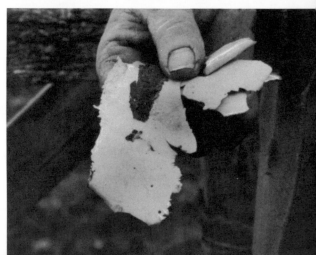

154

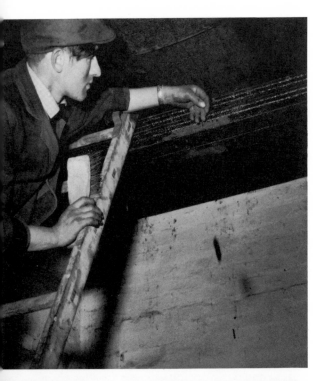

cause it takes a long time for a good-quality paint to start peeling, and a calf will rarely persist in licking a hard, smooth surface.

One of the chief sources of lead paint—a source that is often forgotten—is the iron girders that so often form an integral part of the low roof of a calf pen. Usually such girders are coated with a preservative layer of red lead paint and, when this starts to flake, it falls into the troughs or on to the hay and straw. *(Top, left.)*

Symptoms

In some ways, the symptoms of lead poisoning are similar to those of hypomagnesaemia. In fact, in acute cases they are almost identical. *(Bottom, left.)*

In the less acute case, the calf stops eating, shivers and becomes ice cold, especially at its extremities. It may stumble and stagger and flop out just like a hypomagnesaemia case, though close observation will show that the unsteady movement is mostly due to a loss of vision. In other words, blindness is a diagnostic feature of the condition. *(Below.)*

In recovered cases, blindness may persist for several months. In fact, I have seen it persist for two years in feeding cattle

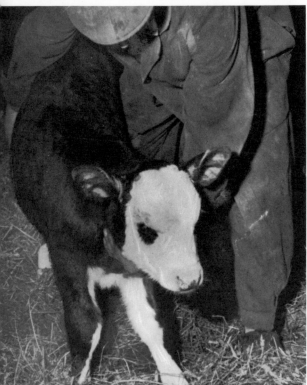

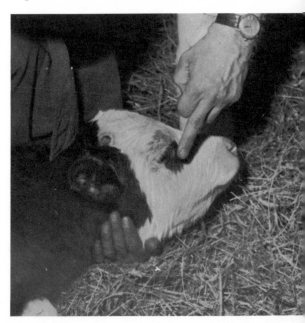

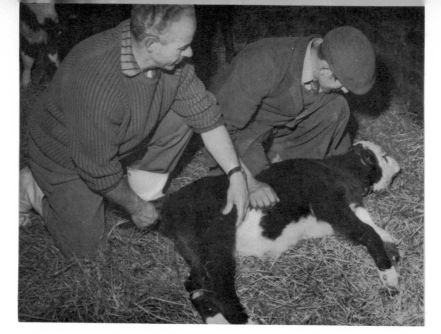

and, occasionally, it can be permanent.

In fatal cases, death is usually preceded by an epileptic-like convulsion. *(Above.)*

What To Do
Any form of treatment is highly unsatisfactory. The toxic effect of the lead often leaves the animal's liver and/or kidneys irrevocably damaged and the blindness, as mentioned above, may be permanent or at least take a long time to get better.

The best first-aid antidote is epsom salts (i.e. magnesium sulphate). In lead poisoning, the epsom salts produces its effect by combining with and inactivating the lead.

The required dose of the epsom salts for a calf is two teaspoonfuls dissolved in water and given as a drench three times daily for at least five days. For an adult animal, up to four ounces can be given twice daily. *(Below, left and right.)*

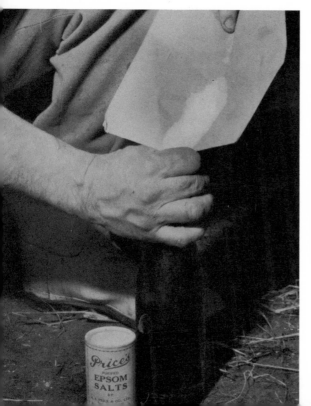

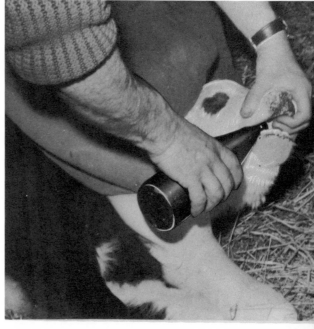

156

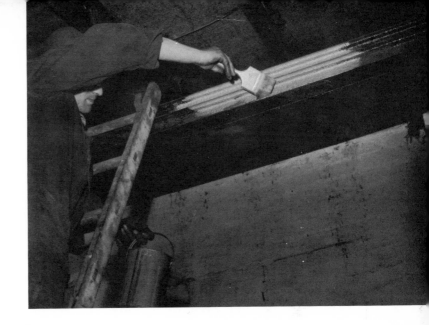

There is a more specific antidote, calcium disodium versenate, but this has to be given intravenously and should only be administered by a veterinary surgeon.

It is wrong to panic into the emergency slaughter of a blind animal, particularly one that can be fattened for the butcher, because it is almost uncanny how the blind cattle adapt themselves to a normal life, finding both trough and water bowl by instinct.

Prevention

So often it is a matter of shutting the stable door after the horse has bolted out. Since treatment is an unsatisfactory compromise, the real answer lies in making sure that you don't get lead poisoning. This is easy. All you have to do is to check your buildings, calf pens, rickyards and pastures for possible sources of lead.

In calf pens, particularly in the older buildings, a priority job must be to burn the paint off any supporting or roof girder and re-coat with non-lead aluminium paint. At the same time, blow-lamp, scrape and repaint all iron beams and the inside doors, again with a lead-free compound. *(Above and left.)*

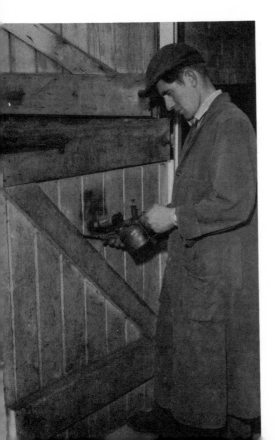

I would say that this should be done in all pens when it is not definitely known whether or not the paint contains lead. The job is not difficult or expensive, it is merely sensible and well worthwhile. The important thing is to make sure from the supplier that the new paint does not contain lead.

Make absolutely certain that none of the herd has access to rubbish dumps or felted fowl pens. In fact, the answer to lead poisoning lies in simple commonsense and good management.

26
Diagnosis at a Glance

The Spastic Calf *(Below.)*
THE typical hind leg movement of a spastic calf, a condition thought to be hereditary. Cases can be operated on successfully by cutting the tendons a few inches above the hock, but the operation is frowned upon by the breed societies.

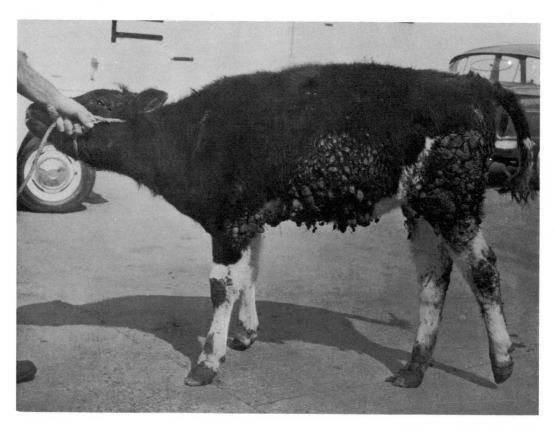

Lice

Lice attack the extremities mainly and a good-going lice infestation will keep your calves from thriving.

As soon as you see a hind end (or fore-end) with the hair being rubbed off, get going with the parasitic dusting powder. It's cheap enough. *(Right.)*

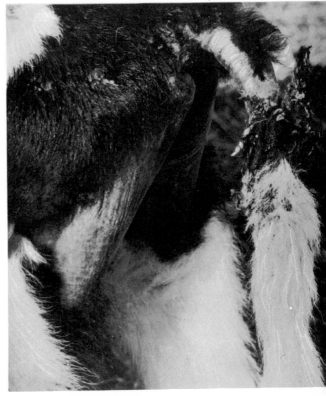

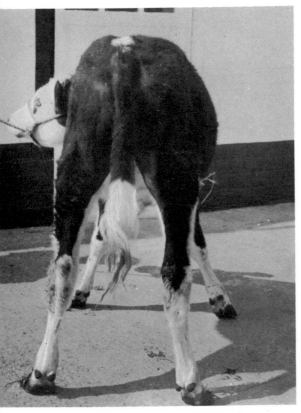

Tetanus (Lockjaw)

Tail cocked up, hind legs splayed, blown on the left flank, and an anxious look in the head—all typical symptoms of tetanus. When made to move backwards, the patient reverses 'all in one piece'.

This is definitely a case for your veterinary surgeon. *(Left.)*

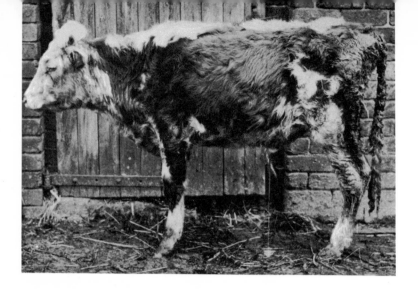

Parasitic Gastro Enteritis

This condition is seen in calves towards the end of the year or, if they have been wintered out during a mild winter, in the early part of the spring.

Hide-bound staring coat, emaciation, sunken eyes, dry mouth, dehydration, and acute anaemia are the symptoms. The anaemia causes the inside of the mouth to look like white paper. *(Above and below.)*

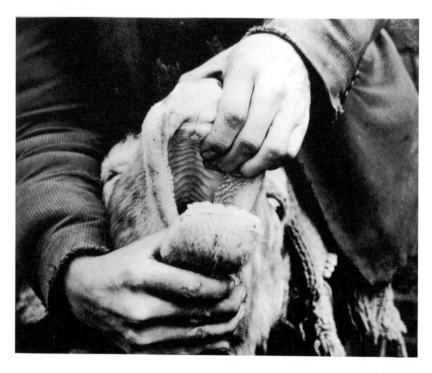

Index